INSTANT NURSING ASSESSMENT:

Cardiovascular

▽   ▽   ▽   ▽   ▽   ▽   ▽

Delmar Publishers' Online Services

To access Delmar on the World Wide Web, point your browser to:
    http://www.delmar.com/delmar.html

To access through Gopher:
    gopher://gopher.delmar.com

(Delmar Online is part of "thomson.com," an Internet site with information on more than 30 publishers of the International Thomson Publishing organization.)

For more information on our products and services:
    email: info@delmar.com or call 800-347-7707

INSTANT NURSING ASSESSMENT:

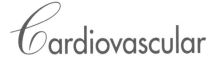

Cardiovascular

▽   ▽   ▽   ▽   ▽   ▽   ▽

Theresa M. O'Neill Korolishin, RNC, MSN
Director, Cardiac Rehabilitation
Nazareth Hospital
Philadelphia, Pennsylvania

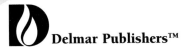 **Delmar Publishers™**

I(T)P™ An International Thomson Publishing Company

Albany • Bonn • Boston • Cincinnati • Detroit • London • Madrid
Melbourne • Mexico City • New York • Pacific Grove • Paris • San Francisco
Singapore • Tokyo • Toronto • Washington

$\mathscr{S}$TAFF

Team Leader:
DIANE McOSCAR

Sponsoring Editors:
PATRICIA CASEY
BILL BURGOWER

Developed for Delmar Publishers by:
JENNINGS & KEEFE Media Development, Corte Madera, CA

Concept, Editorial, and Design Management:
THE WILLIAMS COMPANY, LTD., Collegeville, PA

Project Coordinator:
KATHLEEN LUCZAK

Editorial Administrator:
GABRIEL DAVIS

Production Editor:
BARBARA HODGSON

Manuscript written by:
MARY HUNSCHE
SHARON MARMON-KACZOROWSKI

Text Design:
KM DESIGN GROUP

For information, address:
Delmar Publishers
3 Columbia Circle
Box 15015
Albany, NY 12212-5015

International Thomson Publishing Europe
Berkshire House 168-173
High Holborn
London, WC1V7AA
England

Thomas Nelson Australia
102 Dodds Street
South Melbourne, 3205
Victoria, Australia

Nelson Canada
1120 Birchmount Road
Scarborough, Ontario
Canada M1K 5G4

International Thomson Editores
Campos Eliseos 385, Piso 7
Col Polanco
11560 Mexico D F Mexico

International Thomson Publishing GmbH
Königswinterer Strasse 418
53227 Bonn
Germany

International Thomson Publishing Asia
221 Henderson Road
#05-10 Henderson Building
Singapore 0315

International Thomson Publishing Japan
Hirakawacho Kyowa Building, 3F
2-2-1 Hirakawacho
Chiyoda-ku, Tokyo 102
Japan

Printed in the United States of America
Published simultaneously in Canada
by Nelson Canada, a division of The Thomson Corporation.

1 2 3 4 5 6 7 8 9 10 XXX 00 99 98 97 96 95

Library of Congress Cataloging-in-Publication Data
Korolishin, Theresa M., 1950–
    Instant nursing assessment: cardiovascular/Theresa M.
    Korolishin.
        p. cm. — (Instant nursing assessment)
    Includes bibliographical references and index.
    ISBN 0-8273-7102-0
        1. Cardiovascular system—Diseases—Nursing. I. Title.
    II. Series.
        [DNLM: 1. Nursing Assessment—methods. 2. Nursing
    Assessment—methods. 3. Nursing Diagnosis—methods. 4.
    Cardiovascular Diseases—nursing. WY 152.5 K84i 1995]
    RC674.K67 1995
    610.73' 691—dc20
    DNLM/DLC
    for Library of Congress   95-21007
                                                                CIP

TITLES IN THIS SERIES:

Suzanne K. Marnocha, RN, MSN, CCRN
Assistant Professor, College of Nursing
University of Wisconsin
Oshkosh, Wisconsin

Linda Moody, RN, FAAN, Ph.D.
Professor, Director of Research and Chair,
Gerontology Nursing
College of Nursing
University of South Florida
Tampa, Florida

Patricia A. O'Neill, RN, CCRN, MSN
Instructor, DeAnza College School of Nursing
Cupertino, California

Virgil Parsons, RN, DNSc, Ph.D.
Professor, School of Nursing
San Jose State University
San Jose, California

Elaine Rooney, MSN
Assistant Professor of Nursing, Nursing Department
University of Pittsburgh
Bradford, Pennsylvania

Barbara Shafner, RN, Ph.D.
Associate Professor, Department of Nursing
Otterbein College
Westerville, Ohio

Elaine Souder, RN, Ph.D.
Associate Professor, College of Nursing
University of Arkansas for Medical Sciences
Little Rock, Arkansas

Mary Tittle, RN, Ph.D.
Associate Professor, College of Nursing
University of South Florida
Tampa, Florida

Peggy L. Wros, RN, Ph.D.
Assistant Professor of Nursing
Linfield College School of Nursing
Portland, Oregon

CONTENTS

NOTICE TO THE READER

The publisher, editors, advisors, and reviewers do not warrant or guarantee any of the products described herein nor have they performed any independent analysis in connection with any of the product information contained herein. The publisher, editors, advisors, and reviewers do not assume, and each expressly disclaims, any obligation to obtain and include information other than that provided to them by the manufacturer.

The reader is expressly warned to consider and adopt all safety precautions that might be indicated by the activities described herein and to avoid all potential hazards. By following the instructions contained herein, the reader willingly assumes all risks in connection with such instructions.

The publisher, editors, advisors, and reviewers make no representations or warranties of any kind, including but not limited to the warranties of fitness for particular purpose or merchantability, nor are any such representations implied with respect to the material set forth herein, and the publisher, editors, advisors, and reviewers take no responsibility with respect to such material. The publisher, editors, advisors, and reviewers shall not be liable for any special, consequential, or exemplary damages resulting, in whole or in part, from readers' use of, or reliance upon, this material.

A conscientious effort has been made to ensure that the drug information and recommended dosages in this book are accurate and in accord with accepted standards at the time of publication. However, pharmacology is a rapidly changing science, so readers are advised, before administering any drug, to check the package insert provided by the manufacturer for the recommended dose, for contraindications for administration, and for added warnings and precautions. This recommendation is especially important for new, infrequently used, or highly toxic drugs.

CPR standards are subject to frequent change due to ongoing research. The American Heart Association can verify changing CPR standards when applicable. Recommended Schedules for Immunization are also subject to frequent change. The American Academy of Pediatrics, Committee on Infectious Diseases can verify changing recommendations.

FOREWORD

As quality and cost-effectiveness continue to drive rapid change within the health care system, you must respond quickly and surely—whether you are a student, a novice, or an expert. This *Instant Assessment Series*—and its companion *Nursing Interventions Series*—will help you do that by providing a great deal of nursing information in short, easy-to-read columns, charts, and boxes. This convenient presentation will support you as you practice your science and art and apply the nursing process. I hope you'll come to look on these books as providing "an experienced nurse in your pocket."

The *Instant Assessment Series* offers immediate, relevant clinical information on the most important aspects of patient assessment. The *Nursing Interventions Series* is a handy source for appropriate step-by-step nursing actions to ensure quality care and meet the fast-paced challenges of today's nursing profession. Because more nurses will be working in out-patient settings as we move into the 21st century, these series include helpful information about ambulatory patients.

These books contain several helpful special features, including nurse alerts to warn you quickly about critical assessment findings, nursing diagnoses charts that include interventions and rationales along with collaborative management to help you work with your health care colleagues, patient teaching tips, and the latest nursing research findings.

Each title in the *Instant Assessment Series* begins with a review of general health assessment tools and techniques and then expands to cover a different body system, such as cardiovascular, or a special group of patients, such as pediatric or geriatric. This focused approach allows each book to provide extensive information—but in a quick reference format—to help you grow and excel in your specialty.

Both medical and nursing diagnoses are included to help you adapt to emerging critical pathways, care mapping, and decision trees. All these new guidelines help decrease length of stay and increase quality of care—all current health care imperatives.

I'm confident that each small but powerful volume will prove indispensable in your nursing practice. Each book is formatted to help you quickly connect your assessment findings with the patient's pathophysiology—a cognitive connection that will further help you plan nursing interventions, both independent and collaborative, to care for your patients skillfully and completely. With the help and guidance provided by the books in this series, you will be able to thrive—and survive—in these changing times.

— Helene K. Nawrocki, RN, MSN, CNA
Executive Vice President
The Center for Nursing Excellence
Newtown, Pennsylvania
Adjunct Faculty, La Salle University
Philadelphia, Pennsylvania

SECTION I. GENERAL HEALTH ASSESSMENT REVIEW

Chapter 1. Health History

▽   ▽   ▽   ▽   ▽   ▽   ▽

INTRODUCTION

SEE TEXT PAGES

When taking a health history, collect critical subjective data about the patient. In addition to collecting clues about existing or possible health problems, you are also drawing a road map for future patient interactions. To make this map as useful as possible, gather information about the patient's physical condition and symptoms and explore the patient's psychological, cultural, and psychosocial environment as it pertains to his or her health issues.

BEGINNING CONSIDERATIONS

Collecting vital information about the patient can be a daunting task. Patients are often nervous and apprehensive. They may also feel awkward or embarrassed about sharing their problems and concerns, particularly if they've never seen you before. You may even feel some anxiety about the prospective interview.

You can do several things to ease the situation:
• Create a comfortable physical environment.
• Learn interviewing techniques that will put the patient at ease.

THE EXTERNAL ENVIRONMENT

The external environment is the place where you meet with the patient to collect the health history.

Do the following to help the patient feel at ease:
• Conduct the interview in a quiet, private area.
• Set the thermostat at a comfortable level.
• Make sure the lighting is adequate.
• Avoid interruptions.
• Remove objects that might upset or distract the patient.
• Position yourself and the patient as equals by:
  - Sitting in comfortable chairs at eye level. Standing implies that you are more powerful.
  - Not interviewing the patient from behind a desk or table.

- Maintain an appropriate distance between you and the patient. Be sensitive to cultural differences and the need for personal space.

COMMUNICATING WITH YOUR PATIENT

Successful communication requires good interpersonal skills that place the patient at ease. To do so, use the techniques suggested by the acronym DEAR:
- Demonstrate acceptance
- Empathize openly
- Affirm
- Recognize

The best way to show a patient that you accept what he or she is saying is to listen. People know that you are listening when you make comments like "I see what you are saying" or simply, "I understand." When you nod your head yes and make eye contact, you also show that you are attentive and accepting of what you hear. Acceptance is not the same as believing the patient's statements are right or wrong.

Empathy is the uniquely human ability to put yourself in someone else's shoes, to show that you can relate to his or her feelings. You show empathy when you say such things as "That must have made you sad/frightened/happy/relieved."

When you affirm and recognize, you are putting acceptance and empathy to work. Affirmation is the act of acknowledging what the patient is telling you.

Recognition is listening well and attentively, thus showing the patient by what you say and how you say it that you hear him or her. It can be as simple as nodding yes or saying "Please continue."

Some patients will come to you with as many concerns about the treatment process and environment as about their health. Reassure them that all communication is confidential and that you cannot legally reveal anything beyond the confines of the health care team without the patient's consent.

ℰNSURING A SUCCESSFUL INTERVIEW

Sometimes patients are so apprehensive or have had such negative health care experiences that they are hostile. To best handle such a patient, follow these guidelines:

- Remain calm.
- Never argue with the patient.
- Affirm and recognize his or her feelings using simple sentences.
- Reschedule the interview if the patient's hostility persists.
- If you feel physically intimidated by the patient, call for assistance.

A second factor that can skew the results of your interview is a cultural or ethnic difference between you and the patient. Differences between cultures can be subtle. For example, in the United States, most people consider it rude not to make eye contact. Culturally, the absence of eye contact suggests disinterest or dishonesty. In many other cultures, it is considered extremely rude to make eye contact with elders or authority figures, or eye contact is not made between unrelated members of the opposite sex.

While it is important to be sensitive to cultural differences, try not to go to the other extreme and resort to stereotyping. Each of us is a unique individual regardless of our culture. No one perfectly embodies all the characteristics of a culture.

Sometimes we use the term "ethnic group" to refer to a group that shares a common culture. At other times we use the same term to refer to a group that shares a common biological origin. On still other occasions we use the term to refer to a group that shares a common national origin. Beware of making judgments about a patient's behavior based on biological ethnicity. Skin color is not a good predictor of cultural affiliation. People who are "American" come in all sizes, shapes, and colors.

Pay attention to how culture and individual character affect the patient's lifestyle, fears and hopes about his or her health, and feelings about treatment. This can be an exciting journey for both of you.

The Interview: Your Role

The interview involves two persons—you and the patient—and is really the sum of what both of you bring to it. You, however, are the authority figure, and most patients will expect you to set the tone and direction of the interview. Your goal is to help the patient become a willing participant in his or her own care—to actively assist in discovering solutions to problems he or she may experience. The more you know about successful interviewing techniques, the more likely you are to be at ease with the patient. Remember: These techniques are general guidelines. You are the best judge of what is most effective in any given situation.

Like a college essay, the interview can be broken into three parts: the introduction, the main body (the interview), and the conclusion (parting with the patient).

The Introduction

The introductory phase of the interview sets the tone for the rest of the assessment. It's also where you begin to build a rapport with the patient.
- Always start the interview by introducing yourself and giving the patient some background on your place in the organization. It may help to shake hands. Always ask the patient how he or she likes to be addressed.
- Take a little time to get to know the patient by talking informally before you begin the interview process.

NURSE ALERT:
Make sure the patient speaks fluent English. If not, you may want to postpone the interview until you can obtain an interpreter.

- Explain how long the interview will take.
- Describe the interview process and ask the patient for questions.
- If you need to take notes to remember information, tell the patient you will be doing so in order to listen more attentively.

The Interview

The main body of the interview is where you collect the information you need for the patient's treatment and care. Provide a road map. Begin the interview process by asking general questions. Ask the patient why he or she came in for today's visit. During the interview, help the patient by asking questions such as "Is there anything else you're worried about?"

Repeat important points the patient makes. You can make a comment such as "You just said that your pain occurs early in the morning. Let's explore that for a second."

Another way to draw the road map is to interpret what the patient has said and done. You could say, "It sounds like whenever you are short of breath, something has happened to make you anxious." Clarify the patient's statement as much as possible.

In other situations, the patient may have trouble verbalizing his or her concerns. In this case, a response like "It seems to me that you are concerned about..." shows that you will do whatever is necessary to help the patient communicate more clearly.

Finally, you can help the patient be clear by summarizing major points with statements such as "So far, we've talked about...I think we are ready to go on to talk about...."

Give the patient time to think about what he or she needs to say. This shows that you respect the patient's thought process. Use silence to focus on the patient's nonverbal behavior.

Be an observer. Be aware of the patient's unspoken behavior. When appropriate, use these observations for clarification and to heighten the patient's awareness. Simple observations such as "It appears that that must have been a painful experience" often open new avenues for exploration and discovery.

Affirm the patient's role in the interview as a participant. For example, ask the patient to offer strategies for dealing with his or her health care issues.

Sometimes patients may make statements or have expectations that are unrealistic. Respond by pointing out the obvious—"You told me your side doesn't bother you, but you wince every time I touch it." Or you might say, "You'll feel much better after treatment, but you won't be able to go back to long-distance running."

It is very important that the patient remain grounded. Comments such as "You look worried," "You seem tense," and "You sound more relaxed" affirm the patient's feelings.

You can empower patients to be willing participants in the interview process by openly sharing whatever information and facts you have about their health care and the decisions involved in it. Clearly explain patient care and how the health care system works.

AVOIDING PITFALLS

Just as there are good techniques for interviewing, there are techniques to avoid because they increase tension and reduce communication between you and the patient.

- Justification. When you ask patients how or why something happened, you are implying that they need to explain or defend their behavior. You can also make a patient feel you expect an explanation when you ask leading questions. A leading question always implies that there is a single "right" answer. For example, "You don't eat a lot of fried foods, do you?" is likely to get a no from even the most dedicated french-fry eater.
- Too persistent. There is an old saying about not beating a dead horse that applies to interviews. If you don't get the desired information after a couple of tries, move on.
- The wrong tone. Be careful to gear your discussion to the patient's ability to understand it. On the one hand, don't overwhelm the patient with technical terms and medical jargon. On the other hand, don't talk down to the patient.

Pay attention to how the patient prefers to be addressed. For example, an older woman may find it patronizing and rude if you address her by her first name.

If you are talking about death, use statements such as "he died," not "he's gone to his reward." Pay attention to such euphemisms when used by the patient. They are a way to avoid real feelings, and we most often resort to them when talking about subjects that make us feel anxious or frightened.

Be personable but not personal. If you begin to share your own experiences or provide advice, you are likely to make the patient feel like a nonparticipant in the health care process.

The patient who asks for advice is demonstrating respect and trust. You can repay that with responses such as "Even if I were in the exact same situation as you, I might not want to do the same thing. What do you think is best for you?"

While touch can be comforting to a patient, too much of it can feel inappropriate. Likewise, be aware of becoming too impersonal. When you assume the posture of an authority figure, you create distance between you and the patient. To say, "I'm the nurse and I know best," even when a patient is clearly doing something destructive like smoking, implies that the patient is inferior to you.

Another way to be too impersonal is to use impersonal language. It is the difference between "That wasn't very clear" and "I don't understand." The first statement removes you from the equation. Also, consider the following:
- Losing touch with reality. Making statements such as "It will all be OK," "Don't worry, you'll be fine," or "Life goes on" may make you feel better, but they don't make the patient feel better. Rather, the patient is likely to feel that you don't care about the impact of his or her illness or that you cannot be trusted to tell the truth.
- Interrupting. If you interrupt the patient or change the subject, you are likely to make the patient feel that you are impatient. The same is true of drawing conclusions too quickly. When you draw all the conclusions, the patient is likely to withhold information or tell you what he or she thinks you want to hear.
- Inappropriate emotion. Inappropriate responses to what the patient says include the following:
  - Don't overly praise the response. If, for example, our french-fry eater said no to your leading question about fried foods and you responded with "That's fantastic. It's great that you're so disciplined," you're not likely to find out what his diet and exercise patterns really are.
  - Don't show disapproval or anger.
  - Don't take the patient too literally. If a patient says he is not afraid of needles but pulls his arm away, shuts his eyes, and grits his teeth, he is clearly apprehensive about injections. It's important that you base your response as much on what the patient does as what the patient says.

PARTING WITH THE PATIENT

How you close the interview is as important as how you open and conduct it. Ask the patient if he or she has any other questions or comments and how he or she feels about the treatment decisions. Summarize the information collected in the interview and any decisions that have been made about future treatment. Make sure you and the patient understand this in the same way.

NONVERBAL CUES

Not all communication is spoken. In fact, the majority of communication is nonverbal. You can learn to send nonverbal messages to your patient that emphasize the qualities of DEAR discussed earlier in this chapter.

- Appearance. Be appropriately professional. Avoid dressing in a way that makes the patient uncomfortable.
- Posture. Be relaxed. Keep your arms uncrossed to convey openness. Direct your body toward your patient. Don't slouch.
- Gestures. Occasionally, you can use your hands to encourage conversation. Touch the patient's arm for comfort. Never point at the patient, clench your fist, or drum your fingers. Avoid looking at your watch. Never touch the patient in a way that he or she may find inappropriate.
- Facial expression. Try to look actively interested. Smile and show concern when appropriate. Avoid yawning, which expresses boredom. Try not to frown, grimace, or chew on your lip or cheek. Maintain appropriate eye contact.
- Speech. Keep your voice moderate. Raise it only if the patient has trouble hearing. Watch your tone of voice with patients who speak English as a second language. We all have a tendency to yell when trying to make ourselves understood. Make sure you are not speaking too quickly or too slowly.

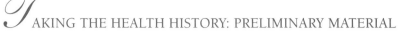

AKING THE HEALTH HISTORY: PRELIMINARY MATERIAL

Having laid out the structure of the interview, it is now time to get down to specifics. Each institution has its own form. Be complete in filling out the form specific to your institution. The table that follows lists initial information you should obtain from your patient.

NURSE ALERT:

If the patient is feeling ill, begin by collecting the relevant information about his or her illness. Collect other information afterward or reschedule the patient. Don't tax the patient's energy with the interview.

HEALTH HISTORY CHECKLIST

AREA TO COVER	SPECIFIC QUESTIONS
Biographical information	Use the form your institution provides.
Allergies	Are you allergic to any: • medications (include reaction) • foods (include reaction) • environmental agents (include reaction)
Medication	What medications (including dosages) do you take on a regular basis? Include both prescription and over-the-counter medications.
Childhood illnesses	Have you had measles, mumps, rubella, chicken pox, pertussis, strep throat, rheumatic fever, scarlet fever, poliomyelitis?
Accidents or injuries	Describe and include dates of any accidents or injuries you've had.
Chronic illnesses	Do you have diabetes, hypertension, heart disease, sickle cell anemia, cancer, AIDS, seizure disorder?

HEALTH HISTORY CHECKLIST *(CONTINUED)*

AREA TO COVER	SPECIFIC QUESTIONS
Hospitalizations	Describe, including dates and diagnoses, any hospitalizations.
Surgical procedures	Describe, with dates and diagnoses, any operations.
Obstetric	How many times have you been pregnant? How many full-term pregnancies have you had? Have you had any abortions?
Immunizations	Did you receive the complete battery of childhood immunizations? What is the date of your most recent tetanus shot, hepatitis B vaccine, tuberculin skin test, flu shot?
Last examination	When were your most recent physical, dental, and eye examinations; hearing test; ECG; and chest X-ray performed?

PHYSIOLOGICAL ASSESSMENT: GENERAL

The following table lists general physiological questions to ask the patient. If the patient is not feeling well, go on to the table titled "Current Complaint." If possible, also cover the family history information listed in the "Family Environment" table.

AREA TO COVER	SPECIFIC QUESTIONS
Present health status	Have you had any recent weight gain or loss? Do you know the cause? Do you experience any of the following? • fatigue, weakness, or malaise • difficulty in carrying out daily activities • fever or chills • sweats or night sweats • frequent colds or other infections Are you able to exercise?
Skin	Do you have a history of any of the following: • eczema, psoriasis, or hives • changes in pigment • changes in any moles • overly dry skin • overly moist skin • excessive bruising • pruritus • rashes • lesions • reaction to heat or cold • itching • sun exposure and amount Describe the location of any growths, moles, tumors, warts, or other skin abnormalities.

PHYSIOLOGICAL ASSESSMENT: GENERAL *(CONTINUED)*

AREA TO COVER	SPECIFIC QUESTIONS
Hair	Describe any recent hair loss, change in hair texture, or change in hair characteristics. How often do you shampoo your hair? Is your hair color-treated or permed? How often do you have this done?
Nails	Have you experienced any of the following: • changes in nail color • changes in nail texture • occurrences of nail splitting, cracking, or breaking • changes in nail shape
Head and neck	Have you experienced any of the following: • frequent or severe headaches • dizziness • pain or stiffness • a head injury • abnormal range of motion • surgery • enlarged glands • vertigo • lumps, bumps, or scars
Eyes	Have you been troubled by any of the following? • eye infections or trauma • eye pain • redness or swelling • change in vision

PHYSIOLOGICAL ASSESSMENT: GENERAL *(CONTINUED)*

AREA TO COVER	SPECIFIC QUESTIONS
Eyes *(continued)*	Have you been troubled by any of the following? • eye infections or trauma • eye pain • redness or swelling • change in vision • spots or other disturbances of the visual field • twitching or other sensations • strabisimus or amblyopia • itching, tearing, or discharge • double vision • glaucoma • cataracts • blurred vision, blind spots, or decreased visual acuity Do you wear glasses? Do you have a history of retinal detachment? When did you last have a glaucoma test and what was the result?
Ears	Have you experienced any of the following? • ear infections or earaches (include dates and frequency) • hearing loss • tinnitus (ringing or crackling) • exposure to environmental noise • discharge from the ear—color, frequency, and amount • vertigo • unusual sensitivity to noise • sensation of fullness in the ears When did you last have an ear examination? What was the result? What impact does your hearing loss have on your daily activities? How do you clean your ears?

PHYSIOLOGICAL ASSESSMENT: GENERAL *(CONTINUED)*

AREA TO COVER	SPECIFIC QUESTIONS
Nose	Do you have a history of the following? • nosebleeds • nasal obstruction • frequent sneezing episodes • nasal drainage—color, frequency, and amount • trauma or fracture to the nose or sinuses • sinus infection (include treatment received) • allergies • postnasal drip • pain over sinuses • change in the sense of smell • difficulty breathing through nose
Mouth and throat	Do you have a history of the following? • oral herpes infections • mouth pain • difficulty chewing or swallowing • lesions in mouth or on tongue • tonsillectomy • altered taste • sore throat (include dates and frequency) • bleeding gums • toothache • hoarseness or change in voice • dysphagia When did you last have a dental examination? What were the results? What is your daily dental care regiment? Do you wear dentures or any other type of dental appliance?

PHYSIOLOGICAL ASSESSMENT: GENERAL *(CONTINUED)*

AREA TO COVER	SPECIFIC QUESTIONS
Respiratory system	Do you have a history of any of the following? • asthma • bronchitis • tuberculosis • shortness of breath-if so, preceded by how much and what type of activity • coughing up blood • noisy breathing • pollution or toxin exposure • emphysema • pneumonia • chronic cough • chest pain with breathing • wheezing • smoking How much sputum do you cough up per day? What color is it?
Cardiovascular system	Have you experienced any of the following? • chest pain • heart murmur • need to be upright to breathe, especially at night • swelling in arms or legs • hair loss on legs • anemia • cramping pain in the legs and feet • leg ulcers • palpitations • color changes in fingers or toes • coronary artery disease • varicose veins • thrombophlebitis • coldness, numbness, or tingling in the fingers or toes Do you have hypertension, high cholesterol levels, or a family history of heart failure? Do you smoke? How many packs per day?

PHYSIOLOGICAL ASSESSMENT: GENERAL (CONTINUED)

AREA TO COVER	SPECIFIC QUESTIONS
Cardiovascular system (continued)	Do you sit or stand for long periods? Do you cross your knees when sitting? Do you use support hose?
Urinary tract	Do you have a history of any of the following? • painful urination • difficulty or hesitancy in starting urine flow • urgency • flank pain • cloudy urine • incontinence • frequent urination at night • pain in suprapubic region • changes in urine • decreased or excessive urine output • kidney stones • blood in the urine • pain in groin • bladder, kidney, or urinary tract infections • low back pain • prostate gland infection or enlargement
Gastrointestinal system	Have you experienced any of the following? • appetite changes • dysphagia • indigestion or pain associated with eating (obtain symptoms) • vomiting blood • ulcers • gallbladder disease • colitis • constipation • black stools • hemorrhoids • food intolerance • heartburn

PHYSIOLOGICAL ASSESSMENT: GENERAL *(CONTINUED)*

AREA TO COVER	SPECIFIC QUESTIONS
Gastrointestinal system *(continued)*	• burning sensation in stomach or esophagus • other abdominal pain • chronic or acute nausea and vomiting • abdominal swelling • liver disease • appendicitis • flatulence • diarrhea • rectal bleeding • fistula How often do you have a bowel movement? Have there been any changes in the characteristics of your stool? Do you use any digestive aids or laxatives? What kind and how often? **THE ELDERLY:** For patients over age 50, obtain the date and results of last Hemoccult test.
Male reproductive system	Do you have a history of any of the following? • penile or testicular pain • penile discharge • hernia • sexually transmitted disease • sores or lesions • penile lumps • prostate gland problems • infertility How often do you perform testicular self-examination? Are you satisfied with your sexual performance? Do you practice safe sex?

PHYSIOLOGICAL ASSESSMENT: GENERAL *(CONTINUED)*

AREA TO COVER	SPECIFIC QUESTIONS
Female reproductive system	Do you have a history of any of the following? • excessive menstrual bleeding • painful intercourse • vaginal itching • bleeding between periods • missed periods • infertility • painful menstruation Provide the following information: • menstrual history, including age of onset, duration, amount of flow, any menopausal signs or symptoms, age at onset of menopause, any postmenopausal bleeding • satisfaction with sexual performance • date of last period • understanding of sexually transmitted disease prevention, including AIDS • number of pregnancies, miscarriages, abortions, stillbirths • date and results of last Pap test • contraceptive practices • vaginal discharge and characteristics **THE ELDERLY:** Ask elderly patients if they have experienced vaginal dryness or other problems.

PHYSIOLOGICAL ASSESSMENT: GENERAL *(CONTINUED)*

AREA TO COVER	SPECIFIC QUESTIONS
Breasts	Have you experienced any of the following? • nipple changes • nipple discharge—color, frequency, odor, amount • rash • breast pain, tenderness, or swelling Have you ever breast-fed? When was your last breast examination? What were the results? Do you perform breast self-examination? When did you last have a mammogram? What were the results? (for women over age 40)
Neurologic system	Do you have a history of any of the following? • seizure disorder, stroke, fainting, or blackouts • weakness, tic, tremor, or paralysis • numbness or tingling • memory disorder, recent or past • speech or language dysfunction • nervousness • mood change • mental health dysfunction • disorientation • hallucinations • depression Do any of these problems affect your day-to-day activities?
Musculoskeletal system	Do you have a history of any of the following? • arthritis or gout • joint or spine deformity • noise accompanying joint motion • fractures • joint pain, stiffness, redness, or swelling (include location, any migration, time of day, and duration)

PHYSIOLOGICAL ASSESSMENT: GENERAL *(CONTINUED)*

AREA TO COVER	SPECIFIC QUESTIONS
Musculoskeletal system *(continued)*	• other pain (include location and any migration) • problems with gait • limitations in motion • muscle pain, cramps, or weakness • chronic back pain or disk disease • problems running, walking, or participating in sports Do any of these problems affect your day-to-day activities?
Immune system	Do you have a history of any of the following? • anemia • low platelet count • blood transfusions (include any reactions) • chronic sinusitis • conjunctivitis • unexplained swollen glands • bleeding tendencies, particularly of skin or mucous membranes • HIV exposure • excessive bruising • fatigue • allergies, hives, itching • frequent sneezing • exposure to radiation or toxic agents • frequent, unexplained infections Do any of these problems affect your day-to-day activities?

PHYSIOLOGICAL ASSESSMENT: GENERAL *(CONTINUED)*

AREA TO COVER	SPECIFIC QUESTIONS
Endocrine system	Do you have a history of any of the following? • excessive urine output • unexplained weakness • changes in hair distribution • hormone therapy • nervousness • inability to tolerate heat or cold • endocrine disease, for example, thyroid or adrenal gland problems, diabetes • increased food intake • excessive thirst • goiter • excessive sweating • tremors • unexplained changes in height or weight • changes in skin pigmentation or texture (In addition discuss the relationship between the patient's weight and appetite.)

PHYSIOLOGICAL ASSESSMENT: CURRENT COMPLAINT

> The following table provides a guide to collecting data about the patient's current complaint. Always begin by having the patient describe, in his or her own words, the reason for today's visit.

AREA TO COVER	SPECIFIC QUESTIONS
Time frame	When did the discomfort or alteration in pain start? Is it intermittent or constant? Is it worse at certain times of day?
Location	Where is the pain located? (Have the patient show you.)
Quality	Describe the pain. Is it sharp or dull? How severe is it?

PHYSIOLOGICAL ASSESSMENT: CURRENT COMPLAINT *(CONTINUED)*

AREA TO COVER	SPECIFIC QUESTIONS
Environment	Are there specific places or activities that seem to trigger the pain? Does anything relieve the pain? Make it worse?
Perception	What do you think your symptoms mean?

ASSESSING FUNCTIONAL STATUS

In addition to collecting specific physiological data, you need to assess the patient's ability to function on a day-to-day basis. The table below provides guidelines for such an assessment.

AREA TO COVER	SPECIFIC QUESTIONS
Daily activities	• What do you do during an average day? Does your complaint interfere with this? If so, in what way? • Do you exercise? If so, what type of exercise do you perform and how often do you exercise? Does your complaint interfere with exercise? If so, in what way? • Do you use street drugs? If so, how often? How has this affected you in terms of work and family?
Sleep and rest	• How long do you sleep? Need to sleep? • Do you have any difficulty falling asleep or staying asleep? • Do you wake during the night to urinate? How often? • Do you feel rested each morning? • Do you feel tired during the day?

ASSESSING FUNCTIONAL STATUS (CONTINUED)

AREA TO COVER	SPECIFIC QUESTIONS
Nutrition	• What have you had to eat or drink in the past 24 hours? Is this a typical daily diet? • Who buys and prepares food in your family? • Is the family income sufficient for the family food budget? • Does the family eat together? • How much caffeine from coffee, tea, or soda do you drink in a day? • When did you last have an alcoholic beverage? What do you drink and how much? Have you ever had a drinking problem?
Stress factors	• Do you live alone? • Do you know your neighbors? • Is the neighborhood safe or high in crime events? • Can you keep the temperature in the house comfortably warm or cool? • Are safety factors at work or in the home a stress factor? • What stressors would you list as present in your life now and in the past year? • Has anything about this stress level changed? • Have you ever tried anything to relieve stress? How well did it work?

FAMILY AND SOCIAL ASSESSMENT

It's particularly important to explore the patient's family history and relationships. The health history provides important clues about the patient's state of health and about how family relationships affect treatment and care.

FAMILY ENVIRONMENT

The following table provides questions you can ask the patient that will help build a picture of his or her family environment. However, these questions imply a nuclear family structure. If the patient comes from a single-parent, gay, or extended family, you will need to modify them accordingly.

AREA TO COVER	SPECIFIC QUESTIONS
Mortality data on blood relatives	What is the age and health of your living blood relatives (parents, grandparents, siblings)? At what age did other relatives die and what was the cause of death?
Family history	Is there any family history of diabetes, heart disease, high blood pressure, stroke, blood disorders, cancer, sickle cell anemia, arthritis, allergies, obesity, alcoholism, mental illness, seizure disorder, kidney disease, tuberculosis?
Spouse and children	What are the ages and health condition of your spouse and children?
Patient's position within the family (The purpose of these questions is to find out how tasks are divided within families with children and to explore family health promotion, factorsthat are very important to patient care.)	• Are you happy with the set of tasks that you and your partner do as spouses and as parents? • Are there differences of opinion about child-rearing? How do you work out any differences? • Do you work outside the home? How does the family support you in your work? • Who is the primary caretaker of the children or older adults in the family? Are you happy with this arrangement? • Who makes doctor appointments, keeps track of medication schedules, and so on?

FAMILY ENVIRONMENT *(CONTINUED)*

AREA TO COVER	SPECIFIC QUESTIONS
Patient's position within the family *(continued)*	• Are you comfortable with how your children are maturing? Are they learning skills like hygiene, good eating habits, appropriate sleep and rest patterns? • Can family members share or switch tasks? Do they have the skills to do so? • Do you and your children have the same values? • If you are the caretaker, how will your family adjust to your illness?
Patient's views of the economics of the family	• Is your family income adequate to supply its basic needs? • Who makes the money decisions in your family?
Patient's support (These questions will help you understand your patient's social skills, the extent to which the patient has access to a support system, and if the patient is likely to feel isolated and depressed.)	• Do you belong to any clubs or organizations outside the family? What do you enjoy about them? • Whom do you ask for help and advice outside your immediate family? • How do you interact with your co-workers? • What do you like to do with your friends? How often do you get to do it? • Are you happy with your friendships? • What do you know about community agencies that can help you while you are ill and recovering?

FAMILY ENVIRONMENT (CONTINUED)

AREA TO COVER	SPECIFIC QUESTIONS
Patient's perception of family	• What is the place of family in your life? • Does your extended family include close friends? • Does anyone who is not a member of your immediate family live in your home? • How do family members interact? • Do they see each other in a positive light? • How do family members react to each other's needs and wants? Are positive and negative feelings expressed openly? • How does the family handle conflicts?

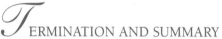

TERMINATION AND SUMMARY

End your interaction with the patient with the following:

- Summarize important information collected during the interview as well as the results of the interview and any conclusions you have drawn from it.
- If there are issues about health education—for example, contraception—either schedule a health education session or provide the patient with the information.
- Make any necessary referrals. Help the patient set up the appointment.
- Summarize decisions you and the patient have made about future care.
- Explain the physical part of the health assessment in detail.
- Ask the patient if he or she has any other concerns or questions.

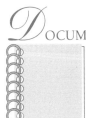

DOCUMENTING THE INTERVIEW

How you document what you have learned from the patient is as important as how you conduct the interview. Other health care professionals will use the patient's record as a basis for future care and treatment. It is important that you allow yourself adequate time to reflect on what the patient has told you and the most effective way to communicate that to other professionals in writing. Observe the following guidelines:

- Use the correct form.
- Use an ink pen, not a pencil.
- Write the patient's name and identification number on each page.
- Make sure the date and time appear with each entry.
- Use standard abbreviations that everyone will understand.
- Wherever possible, use the patient's description of symptoms.
- Wherever possible, be specific, not vague. Do not generalize.
- Do not leave anything blank. If something is not applicable, write "N/A" in that space.
- Do not backdate an entry.
- Never write on a previous entry.
- Never document for anyone but yourself.

Chapter 2. Physical Assessment Skills

▽   ▽   ▽   ▽   ▽   ▽   ▽

Introduction

SEE TEXT PAGES

In the first chapter we explored techniques for the subjective portion of the health history. In this chapter we explore techniques for the objective portion—the physical assessment. This portion of the assessment will either confirm or bring into question the conclusions you and the patient drew during the subjective assessment. It can generate new avenues of exploration.

Tools of the Trade

You yourself provide the most important equipment used in the assessment—your eyes, ears, nose, and fingers. What you see, hear, smell, and touch is critical. You will supplement those tools with special equipment. At a minimum, you will require a measuring tape, penlight or flashlight, thermometer, and visual acuity chart. You will also need additional basic equipment to complete the assessment. (See chart below.)

ASSESSMENT TOOLS

TOOL	USE
Wooden tongue depressor	Assess the patient's gag reflex and obtain a view of the pharynx.
Safety pins	Test the patient's sensation of dull and sharp pain.
Cotton balls	Test the patient's sensation of fine touch.
Test tubes of hot and cold water	Test the patient's ability to distinguish temperature.
Common substances, like coffee or vinegar	Test the patient's ability to smell and taste.

ASSESSMENT TOOLS (CONTINUED)

TOOL	USE
Disposable latex gloves	When handling body fluids (taking blood, rectal, and vaginal assessment)
Water-soluble lubricant	Assess rectum and vagina.

SPECIALIZED ASSESSMENT TOOLS

You may find that you need more specialized equipment to complete your assessment. Such equipment may include one or all of the following: reflex hammer, skin calipers, vaginal speculum, goniometer, transilluminator, ophthalmoscope, nasoscope, otoscope, and tuning fork. These tools require additional training to use correctly.

TOOL	DESCRIPTION	USES
Ophthalmoscope	Light source with a system of lenses and mirrors	Examine the internal eye structure: • Use the large aperture for most patients. • If the patient has small pupils, use the small aperture. • Use the target aperture to localize and measure fundal lesions. • Use the slit beam to measure lesion elevation and the anterior eye. • Use the green filter to determine specific fundal details.

NURSE ALERT:
You can adjust the intensity of light, but it's best to begin at the lowest level to avoid causing discomfort to the patient.

SPECIALIZED ASSESSMENT TOOLS (*CONTINUED*)

TOOL	DESCRIPTION	USES
Otoscope	Light source similar to the ophthalmoscope.	Examine the external auditory canal and tympanic membrane.
Nasoscope	Three types: •Nasal speculum •A speculum for the nostrils that you attach to an ophthalmoscope •Handle like an ophthalmoscope, with short, slim head with light source	Examine the nasal interior. **!** **NURSE ALERT:** If you are not skilled in the use of the nasoscope, do not use it. You can cause the patient discomfort.
Tuning fork	Shaped like a fork. Tines are designed to vibrate.	Check hearing and sensation.

DRAPING AND POSITIONING TECHNIQUES

Before you begin the actual assessment, you need to understand how to position and drape the patient. The correct technique varies, depending on the body area you are assessing. This table provides a quick description of draping and positioning techniques.

BODY AREA	POSITION	DRAPING
Head, neck, and thorax	Patient sits on edge of examination table.	None
Neurologic	In some cases, patient needs to to stand or sit.	None

DRAPING AND POSITIONING TECHNIQUES *(CONTINUED)*

BODY AREA	POSITION	DRAPING
Musculoskeletal	In some cases, patient needs to stand or sit.	None
Breast exam	Phase one: Seated Phase two: Supine, with pillow or towel under the shoulder on the side you are examining; have patient place arm on that side above her head.	None
Abdomen	Supine	Towel over female patient's breasts; for both sexes, sheet draped over lower half of body; do not pull the sheet below the pubic area
Cardiovascular	Supine	Sheet draped over torso and legs
	Sitting	Sheet draped over areas not being auscultated
Rectal (male)	Bent over the examination table or lying on left side	None
Rectal or reproductive (female)	Lithotomy position	Sheet draped over chest and knees and between legs

Assessment Techniques

Palpation

You will use palpation, or different kinds of touch, throughout the assessment. Generally, palpation will follow inspection.

It is particularly important to palpate the abdominal or urinary tract systems at the end of the assessment. Otherwise, you may cause the patient unnecessary discomfort and distort findings.

During the assessment, you are likely to use four types of palpation. Light palpation requires a gentle touch with just the fingertips. Do not indent the skin more than 3/4 in (2 cm). If you push too hard, you will dull the sensation in your fingertips.

Deep palpation is more aggressive and usually involves both hands. Depress the skin 1.5 in (4 cm). Place the opposite hand on top of the palpating hand, using it as a control and guide. Use this technique to locate and examine organs such as the kidney and spleen or to anchor an organ like the uterus with one hand while examining it with the other. A variation on this technique involves using one hand to depress the skin and then removing it quickly. If the patient complains of increased pain as you release pressure, you have discovered an area of rebound tenderness.

NURSE ALERT:

If you use this variation during an examination of the abdomen and the patient feels rebound tenderness, consider the possibility that the patient may have peritonitis.

Light ballottement is a variation on light palpation. Using your fingertips, move from area to area, depressing the skin lightly, but quickly. Be sure to maintain contact with the patient so that you can identify tissue rebound.

Deep ballottement is a variation on deep palpation. Using your fingertips, move from area to area, depressing the skin deeply, but quickly. Be sure to maintain contact with the patient's skin.

Percussion

With percussion, you use your fingertips or hands to tap areas of the patient's body. Tapping can be used to make sounds, to find tender areas, or to judge your patient's reflexes. When used for sound, percussion requires specialized training and the ability to distinguish between slight differences in the sounds produced. Move from areas that make clear sounds to dull areas.

There are three percussion techniques: indirect, direct, and blunt.
- Indirect percussion involves both hands. Place the second finger of your left hand if right-handed or your right hand if left-handed against the appropriate body area—for example, the abdomen. Use the middle finger of your other hand to sharply and quickly tap your finger over the body area just below your first joint. Remember to keep the wrist of the tapping hand loose and relaxed.
- Direct percussion uses the hand or fingertip to directly tap a body area. This method is used to find tender spots and to examine a child's thorax.
- Blunt percussion uses the fist, either directly on the body area or on the back of your opposite hand, which is placed on the body area. You use this method to find tender spots. A second type of blunt percussion involves the use of the reflex hammer to create muscle contraction.

NORMAL AND ABNORMAL PERCUSSION SOUNDS

BODY AREA	SOUND	DESCRIPTION
Healthy lung	Resonance	Long, low, moderate to loud, hollow
Hyperinflated lung	Hyperresonance	Long duration, extremely loud and low-pitched, booming

NORMAL AND ABNORMAL PERCUSSION SOUNDS *(CONTINUED)*

BODY AREA	SOUND	DESCRIPTION
Pleural fluid accumulation or thickening (abnormal)	Dullness	Soft to moderately loud, thud
Abdomen ·	Tympany	Moderate duration, high-pitched, loud drum-like over hollow organs: stomach, intestine, bladder
	Dullness	Moderate duration, high-pitched, soft to moderately loud, thud
		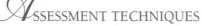 **THE PREGNANT PATIENT:** Liver, full bladder, uterus of pregnant woman
Muscle (normal)	Flatness	Short duration, soft, high-pitched, flat

ASSESSMENT TECHNIQUES

 Auscultation is the process of listening to the sounds different body areas produce—for example, the heart and lungs. You can hear many body sounds, such as the wheeze of the asthma sufferer, with your ear. Other sounds, such as a heart murmur, require the use of a stethoscope. With the exception of the abdomen, auscultation is the last procedure you conduct in the assessment. When assessing the abdomen, first visually inspect it and then listen for sounds. End the assessment with percussion and palpation. Otherwise, bowel sounds may be disrupted by the examination.

When using a stethoscope, observe the following procedure:

- Conduct the exam in a quiet environment.
- Use a quality instrument with bell and diaphragm with ear pieces that fit you comfortably.
- Expose the body area to which you are listening—fabric can obscure sound.
- Remind the patient not to talk during the procedure, and ask the patient to stay as still as possible.
- Warm the stethoscope head with your hand. If it is cold, the patient may jump or shiver, which will result in extraneous sounds.
- Place the stethoscope head over the body area.
- Close your eyes to eliminate any distractions.
- Listen carefully and develop a complete description of any sound you hear, including how often each occurs.

PERFORMING THE ASSESSMENT

In most cases, you will not have the luxury of conducting the entire assessment. In such cases, gear the assessment to the diagnosis. Use the guidelines in Chapter 1, "Health History," when conducting the assessment.

COMPONENTS OF THE ASSESSMENT

A full assessment is based on the patient's health history (see Chapter 1, "Health History"). You end it with an examination of all the body areas. Note any factors, including race, gender, and age, that may affect a diagnosis. Pay attention to any signs of personal distress. Signs of distress include the following:

- shortness of breath—suggesting a respiratory or cardiac problem
- wheezing or difficulty sitting still—suggesting asthma
- labored breathing—suggesting pneumonia or heart failure
- withdrawn posture, arms crossed, rapid speech, sudden hand movements—suggesting emotional distress
- limited movement, grimacing, clutching the affected area—suggesting pain

NURSE ALERT:
For severe pain, especially in the chest or abdomen, you may need to contact a physician immediately.

Assessing Elderly Patients

When assessing elderly patients, it is more important to explore current complaints than collect a past history. You may also need to modify the assessment if your patient appears confused. In that case, ask simple, direct questions and enlist the aid of someone close to the patient. Otherwise, follow the guidelines in this chapter.

Aging may reduce the body's resistance to illness, tolerance of stress, and ability to recuperate from an injury. It can also cause weakening and stiffening of the muscles; loss of hearing, sight, or the ability to smell; slowing of reflexes; and changes in vital signs.

In some cases, aging may mean a loss of intellectual and reasoning skills. Heart disease, diabetes, cataracts, and cancer are more prevalent among older patients.

It's also important to bear in mind that the elderly patient may be on many different medications. You should always watch such a patient for adverse drug reactions and interactions.

When you assess elderly patients, follow these guidelines:
- Always be respectful of the patient. Establish whether or not the patient is comfortable with conversing on a first-name basis.
- Be sure the patient can understand and follow your explanations and instructions. If not, speak slowly and simply.
- Be patient—the elderly patient may take longer to answer your questions or respond to your suggestions.
- Make sure the patient doesn't have a hearing problem. On the other hand, don't automatically raise your voice.
- Some elderly patients may have to move slowly and will have trouble getting from one position to another during the assessment. Allow them extra time.
- Watch for evidence that the patient is beginning to have difficulty taking care of himself or herself.
- Watch for evidence that the patient is not eating properly.
- Learn to identify the symptoms of age-specific diseases, such as osteoporosis and Parkinson's disease.
- Observe the patient for signs of depression. If an ordinarily neat patient begins to show up for appointments in disarray, depression may be the underlying fac-

tor. Depression can also cause mood swings, irritability, and difficulty paying attention.

- If you observe confusion in the patient, do not assume that it results from changes in the brain. Drugs, poor eating habits, dehydration, and even a change in surrounding and routines can all cause confusion in elderly people.
- Maintain a positive attitude toward normal changes of aging.

ASSESSING DISABLED PATIENTS

When assessing disabled patients, make any necessary adjustments. For example, a mute patient should be given a written questionnaire. Or, you may need a sign interpreter for a deaf patient. Use simple, direct sentences and questions with an intellectually impaired patient. In any case, it is helpful to have a close friend or relative attend the visit with the patient.

When assessing such a patient, observe the following:
- Adapt your interaction with the patient to his or her abilities.
- Establish to what extent the patient can be a participant in the assessment before you begin. A severely mentally disabled patient may not be able to participate at all. Other patients may require special assistance.
- Be sensitive to the patient's needs and emotional state.
- Pay attention to the patient's feelings about the disability and about the assessment itself.
- Ascertain the patient's level of independence.

TRANSCULTURAL CONSIDERATIONS

Do not confuse cultural differences with abnormal behavior. Before drawing any conclusions, try to get a feel for cultural differences.

TAKING VITAL SIGNS

The taking of vital signs is fundamental to the physical assessment. Specifically, you check the patient's pulse, respiration, temperature, and blood pressure. Vital signs allow you to establish baseline values for the patient and record changes in the patient's health status. It is preferable to take the signs at once because variations from the norm can indicate possible problems with the patient's health.

A single measure of a vital sign is less reliable than multiple measurements. Ask patients what is normal for them.

If a patient shows an abnormal pattern in a vital sign, make sure that you don't show any apprehension or concern. You should explore any change in vital signs.

NURSE ALERT:
If you take a reading that you think is inaccurate, repeat it. If it still seems inaccurate, have another nurse perform the reading. If you still question the reading, try using a different instrument to check its validity. Explain why you are repeating the measurement.

*M*EASURING HEIGHT AND WEIGHT

Keeping track of your patient's height and weight is as important as assessing his or her vital signs. When measurements are taken regularly, they help you track the patient's growth and development. If, for example, the patient exhibits a sudden weight loss, this alerts you to the possible onset of illness.

You will also use height and weight in calculating doses of drugs. They are also a way of measuring the success of drugs, fluid, or nutrients administered I.V.

*M*EASURING PULSE

To take the pulse, you generally use the wrist. If the patient's wrist is injured, or if the patient has diabetes or vascular insufficiency, you will also check all the peripheral pulses to make sure that circulation is normal.

When taking the pulse, palpate the artery for 60 seconds while applying gentle compression. It's less accurate to count for 15 seconds and multiply by 4 because you are likely to miss any abnormalities in heart rate or rhythm.

NURSE ALERT:
If you must use the carotid artery, be extremely careful with the amount of pressure you place on the artery. Too much pressure can trigger reflex bradycardia. Never press on both carotid arteries at once because you can disrupt circulation to the brain.

When taking an infant's or a toddler's pulse, you can either auscultate the apical pulse or palpate the carotid, femoral, atrial, or brachial pulse. You can also take the pulse by watching the movement of the anterior fontanelle.

ℳEASURING BLOOD PRESSURE

When taking blood pressure, observe the following:

- Check that the patient has not exercised or eaten in the past 30 minutes.
- Make sure that the patient is relaxed.
- Check that the cuff is the right size for the patient. If the cuff is too small, the blood pressure will be falsely elevated; if the cuff is too large, the blood pressure will be falsely lowered.
- Make sure that the bladder is centered over the brachial artery.
- Keep the patient's arm level with the heart by supporting it.
- Listen for pulse sounds as you slowly open the air valve:
  - The beginning of a clear, soft tapping that increases to a thud or loud tap. This is the systolic presssure sound.
  - The change of the tapping to a soft, swishing sound
  - The return of the clear tapping sound
  - A muffled, blowing sound. This is the first diastolic sound. If your patient is a child or physically active adult, this reading is the most accurate reading of diastolic pressure.
  - The disappearance of the muffled, blowing sound. This is the second diastolic sound.

It is more accurate to record the blood pressure readings at the systolic pressure, the first diastolic and the second diastolic sound—for example—110/72/70, although this is not usually done in daily practice.

ASSESSING RESPIRATORY PATTERNS

When assessing respiration, be sure to ascertain the rate, rhythm, and depth.

RESPIRATORY PATTERNS

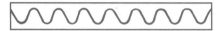

Eupnea
Normal respiratory rate and rhythm

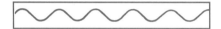

Tachypnea
Increased respiratory rate

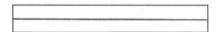

Bradypnea
Slow but regular respirations

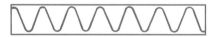

Apnea
Periodic absence of breathing

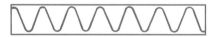

Hyperventilation
Deeper respirations, but at normal rate

ASSESSING REPIRATORY PATTERNS (*CONTINUED*)

RESPIRATORY PATTERNS

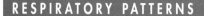

CHEYNE-STOKES
Gradually quickening and deepening respirations, alternating with slower respirations and periods of apnea

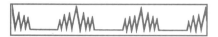

BIOT'S
Faster and deeper than normal respirations of equal depth punctuated with abrupt pauses

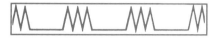

KUSSMAUL'S
Faster and deeper than normal respirations without pauses

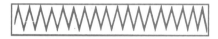

APNEUSTIC
Respirations with prolonged, gasping inspirations followed by very short, inefficient expiration

*C*hapter 3. Head-to-Toe Physical Assessment

▽   ▽   ▽   ▽   ▽   ▽   ▽

*I*NTRODUCTION

SEE TEXT PAGES

This chapter contains a collection of charts that will serve as a guide to assessing the patient from head to toe.

ASSESSMENT TECHNIQUES: HEAD AND NECK

ASSESSMENT	NORMAL FINDINGS	DEVIATIONS FROM NORMAL
Inspect hair, scalp color, and condition.	Normal color; normal texture; full distribution over scalp; scalp pink, smooth, mobile, and free of lesions **THE ELDERLY:** May have thin hair.	Thinning or thickening of the hair—endocrine disorders or side effects from medications; dandruff; dull, coarse, brittle hair; nits
Palpate from the forehead to the posterior triangle of the neck for posterior cervical lymph nodes.	Symmetrical, rounded normocephalic head, positioned at midline, with no lumps or ridges	Note unusual asymmetry, changes in head size, enlarged or painful lymph glands
Palpate around the ears, under the chin, and in the anterior triangle for anterior cervical lymph nodes.	Nonpalpable lymph nodes or small, soft, round, mobile lymph nodes without tenderness	Note the location, size, consistency, tenderness, temperature, and mobility of any enlarged nodes

ASSESSMENT TECHNIQUES: HEAD AND NECK (CONTINUED)

ASSESSMENT	NORMAL FINDINGS	DEVIATIONS FROM NORMAL
Auscultate the carotid arteries.	No bruit on auscultation	Bruit—area of turbulent blood flow
Palpate the trachea.	Straight, midline	Deviation from the midline
Use only one finger to palpate the suprasternal notch.	Palpable pulsations with even rhythm	Abnormal aortic arch pulsations
Palpate the supraclavicular area.	Nonpalpable lymph nodes	Enlarged lymph nodes
Gently palpate the left and then the right carotid artery using the index and middle fingers.	Equal pulse amplitude and rhythm	Unequal pulse amplitude and rhythm

!

NURSE ALERT:
Do not palpate both sides of the anterior neck at the same time. If you accidentally press on both carotid arteries, you may interrupt blood flow to the brain.

ASSESSMENT TECHNIQUES: HEAD AND NECK (CONTINUED)

ASSESSMENT	NORMAL FINDINGS	DEVIATIONS FROM NORMAL
Use the pads of your fingers to palpate the thyroid gland; inside the sternocleidomastoid muscle and below the cricoid and thyroid cartilage.	Thin, mobile thyroid isthmus; non-palpable thyroid lobes	Enlarged or tender thyroid, nodules **!** **NURSE ALERT:** If you find an enlarged thyroid, auscultate for bruits.
Have patient shrug the shoulders against resistance applied by your hands.	Normal range of motion, equal range and strength **THE ELDERLY** May have difficulty tilting the head. Only move the head to the point of discomfort.	Loss of full range of motion
Have patient touch chin to the chest and to each shoulder, touch ear to each shoulder, and tilt head back	Equal strength and movement	Asymmetrical strength or movement
Have patient push left cheek and then right cheek against your hand.	Equal strength and movement	Asymmetrical strength or movement

ASSESSMENT TECHNIQUES: HEAD AND NECK (*CONTINUED*)

ASSESSMENT	NORMAL FINDINGS	DEVIATIONS FROM NORMAL
Inspect patient's face.	Symmetrical facial features	Edema, lesions, or deformities
Have patient smile, wrinkle forehead, puff cheeks.	Symmetrical in all actions	Asymmetrical in any action
Inspect nose.	Symmetrical and non-deviated; tissue pink and nontender	Edema, deformity, nasal discharge, discoloration, flared nostrils, redness, swelling
		! NURSE ALERT: Note color of any mucus.
Alternate holding one nostril shut while patient breathes through the other.	Equal functioning, both passages clear	Inability to breathe through either or both nostrils
Support the patient's head with your free hand and use an ophthalmoscope handle with a nasal attachment to inspect internal nostrils. **!** NURSE ALERT: Don't use an ophthalmoscope handle with a nasal attachment on an infant or young child. It is too sharp. Use a flashlight for illumination instead.	Pink mucosa THE PREGNANT PATIENT: Nasal mucosa may be mildly swollen.	Inflamed, swollen mucosa; polyps

ASSESSMENT TECHNIQUES: HEAD AND NECK (*CONTINUED*)

ASSESSMENT	NORMAL FINDINGS	DEVIATIONS FROM NORMAL
Gently palpate the nose.	Symmetrical, smooth	Edema, bumps, tenderness, asymmetry
Percuss and palpate the sinuses.	No tenderness	Tenderness. If tender, transilluminate the sinuses.

!

NURSE ALERT:
Prior to age 8, the frontal sinus is too small to percuss or palpate.

Have patient open and close mouth while you palpate temporomandibular joints with your middle three fingers.	Smooth, quiet movement; bones aligned	Misalignment, tenderness, clicking

ASSESSMENT TECHNIQUES: HEAD AND NECK *(CONTINUED)*

ASSESSMENT	NORMAL FINDINGS	DEVIATIONS FROM NORMAL
Inspect interior structure of mouth with tongue depressor and penlight.	Pink mucosa and gingiva	Inflammation, edema

NURSE ALERT:
Have the patient remove any dental prosthetics. Wear gloves.

THE PREGNANT PATIENT
In the pregnant patient, you may find the gingiva to be swollen.

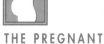

TRANSCULTURAL CONSIDERTIONS:
The mucosa of dark-skinned patients is bluish. This pigmentation is normal.

THE CHILD
A child may have as many as 20 baby teeth. The emergence of baby teeth begins at approximately 6 months. Baby teeth are replaced by secondary teeth between the ages of 6 and 12.

ASSESSMENT TECHNIQUES: HEAD AND NECK (CONTINUED)

ASSESSMENT	NORMAL FINDINGS	DEVIATIONS FROM NORMAL
Inspect the tongue and palates. **NURSE ALERT:** Use this to check hydration in children.	Pink, moist; without ulcers or lesions	Inflammation; lesions; dry, cracked tongue; coated tongue; red inflamed tongue; gingiva on palate
Have patient stick out tongue.	Midline	Cannot hold tongue straight
Have patient stick out tongue and say "Ahh."	Soft palate and uvula rise symmetrically; pink, midline uvula; both tonsils behind pillars	Asymmetry of structures; swollen, inflamed tonsils
Lightly touch back of tongue to test gag reflex. **NURSE ALERT:** If your patient is nauseated, you may want to skip this assessment.	Patient gags; if swallowing is intact, usually gag reflex is present	No gag reflex **NURSE ALERT:** Perform when problem suspected with cranial nerves 9 and 10.

ASSESSMENT TECHNIQUES: HEAD AND NECK (*CONTINUED*)

ASSESSMENT	NORMAL FINDINGS	DEVIATIONS FROM NORMAL
Have patient push against tongue depressor with each side of tongue.	Symmetrical movement and strength	Asymmetry, loss of taste **NURSE ALERT:** If patient reports loss of taste, test with cotton swabs dipped in vinegar, sugar, etc.
Use a test tube containing a familiar substance, like coffee, to test smell. **NURSE ALERT:** Have patient close eyes.	Correctly identifies substance	Unable to identify common substance
Test visual acuity using Snellen eye chart. **THE CHILD:** A young child's vision may be 20/30.	20/20 vision; patients over age 40 may have reduced near vision.	Hesitancy, squinting, vision poorer than 20/30—suggest patient visit an ophthalmologist

ASSESSMENT TECHNIQUES: HEAD AND NECK (CONTINUED)

ASSESSMENT	NORMAL FINDINGS	DEVIATIONS FROM NORMAL
Have patient read newsprint aloud held at a distance of 12 to 14 in (30.5 to 35.5 cm)	Normal near vision	Abnormal near vision—suggest patient visit an ophthalmologist

NURSE ALERT:
Make sure patient wears any corrective lenses.

NURSE ALERT:
If patient is illiterate, use Snellen E chart.

| Have patient identify pattern of colored dots on a special color plate. | Identifies pattern; accurate color perception | Cannot identify pattern |

NURSE ALERT:
It's very important to diagnose color blindness in a child as early as possible. This gives the child ample time to learn to compensate and alerts parents and other caretakers.

ASSESSMENT TECHNIQUES: HEAD AND NECK (CONTINUED)

ASSESSMENT	NORMAL FINDINGS	DEVIATIONS FROM NORMAL
Perform six cardinal positions of gaze test.	Bilaterally equal eye movement; no nystagmus	Nystagmus **!** **NURSE ALERT:** Refer any patient who cannot pass this test to an ophthamlologist.
Perform cover/uncover test.	Eyes steady; no jerking or wandering eye movement	Wandering, jerking **!** **NURSE ALERT:** Refer any patient who cannot pass this test to an ophthalmologist.
Perform corneal light reflex test.	Eyes steadily fixed on an object Bilateral corneal light reflection	Eyes not parallel when fixed on an object **!** **NURSE ALERT:** Refer any patient who cannot pass this test to an ophthalmologist.

ASSESSMENT TECHNIQUES: HEAD AND NECK *(CONTINUED)*

ASSESSMENT	NORMAL FINDINGS	DEVIATIONS FROM NORMAL
Test peripheral vision.	Normal vision laterally, above, down, and medially, **THE ELDERLY** Patient may have decreased peripheral vision.	Vision deviates from 50 degrees from top, 60 degrees medially, 70 degrees downward, 110 degrees laterally; detects only large defects in peripheral vision
Inspect external eye structures.	Clear, symmetrical eyes; even eyelashes **THE ELDERLY** May have few eyelashes, dull eyes. **TRANSCULTURAL CONSIDERATIONS** Asian patients may have eyelids with epicanthal folds.	Cloudy eyes with nystagmus, asymmetry, lid lag, bulging, edema, redness, outward or inward-turning lids, styes, edema, scaling, lesions, unequally distributed eyelashes, eyelashes curve inward, reddened lacrimal apparatus

ASSESSMENT TECHNIQUES: HEAD AND NECK (CONTINUED)

ASSESSMENT	NORMAL FINDINGS	DEVIATIONS FROM NORMAL
Palpate lacrimal apparatus to check tear ducts.	Nontender, pink; without drainage or lumps	Tenderness, masses, too much tearing, drainage

NURSE ALERT:
Culture any drainage.

Examine conjunctiva and sclera.	Pink conjunctiva with no drainage; clear sclera	Edema, drainage, hyperemic blood vessels, inflammation, conjunctivitis, color changes in sclera, scleral icterus

NURSE ALERT:
Wash hands between examining each eye.

THE ELDERLY
May have pinguecula.

TRANSCULTURAL CONSIDERATIONS
Small spots on sclera are normal in dark-skinned patients.

ASSESSMENT TECHNIQUES: HEAD AND NECK (CONTINUED)

ASSESSMENT	NORMAL FINDINGS	DEVIATIONS FROM NORMAL
Shine penlight across eye to examine cornea, iris, and anterior chamber.	Clear, transparent **THE ELDERLY** Cornea may have thin, graying ring. **TRANSCULTURAL CONSIDERATIONS** A gray-blue cornea is normal in dark-skinned patients.	Clouding of cornea, portion of iris does not illuminate
Check pupils.	PERRLA: pupils equal, round, reactive to light and accommodation **THE ELDERLY** After age 85 pupils may not react to accommodation.	Asymmetry in size, asymmetrical reaction to light or its absence, fixed pupils, dilated or constricted pupils
Use ophthalmoscope to check red reflex.	Clearly defined orange-red glow	Absence of red reflex—indicative of opacity and clouding

ASSESSMENT TECHNIQUES: HEAD AND NECK *(CONTINUED)*

ASSESSMENT	NORMAL FINDINGS	DEVIATIONS FROM NORMAL
Check ears.	Line up with eyes, same color as face, symmetrical and proportional to face	Asymmetry, lesions, redness, hard-packed ear wax, drainage, nodules

THE ELDERLY
Reduced adipose tissue and hardened cartilage

TRANSCULTURAL CONSIDERATIONS
Ear wax is yellow in light-skinned patients and dark orange or brown in dark-skinned patients.

Palpate ear and mastoid process.	Absence of pain, tenderness, and swelling	Tenderness, pain, edema, lesions, nodules

NURSE ALERT:
If otitis externa, tenderness, or edema is present, be careful with the otoscope—you may be unable to use it.

ASSESSMENT TECHNIQUES: HEAD AND NECK (*CONTINUED*)

ASSESSMENT	NORMAL FINDINGS	DEVIATIONS FROM NORMAL
Check hearing in each ear by whispering or holding a ticking watch to the ear.	Normal hearing (whisper from 1 to 2 ft; tick from 5 in) **!** **NURSE ALERT:** Note the distance at which you perform the test.	Loss of hearing
Weber's test with tuning fork.	Vibrations heard equally in both ears	Sound heard best in ear with conductive hearing loss
Rinne test with tuning fork.	Equal period of hearing in front of ear and on mastoid process	Conductive or sensorineural hearing loss; vibrations heard longer on mastoid process or front of ear

ASSESSMENT TECHNIQUES: POSTERIOR THORAX

ASSESSMENT	NORMAL FINDINGS	DEVIATIONS FROM NORMAL
Examine the back.	Normal skin tone, symmetry of structure, shoulder height, and inhalation	Asymmetry, accessory muscle use, scoliosis

ASSESSMENT TECHNIQUES: POSTERIOR THORAX (CONTINUED)

ASSESSMENT	NORMAL FINDINGS	DEVIATIONS FROM NORMAL
Examine the antero-posterior and lateral thorax.	2:1 relationship between lateral and anteroposterior diameter	Increased diameter indicative of pul-monary disease
THE CHILD Measure chest cir-cumference at nip-ples.	**THE ELDERLY** Diameter ratio may normally increase.	
Palpate the spine.	Straight alignment Firm, symmetrical	Abnormal alignment, lesions, tenderness, asymmetrical muscles, pain
Palpate the posterior thorax.	Normal, smooth	Lesions, lumps, pain, inflammation, abnor-malities
Percuss the cos-tovertebral area.	Normal thud	Pain, tenderness

ASSESSMENT TECHNIQUES: POSTERIOR THORAX (CONTINUED)

ASSESSMENT	NORMAL FINDINGS	DEVIATIONS FROM NORMAL
Inspect respiratory function.	Symmetrical expansion and contraction	Asymmetry
Palpate as patient says "99" over and over.	Symmetrical vibration Note: Vibration varies over chest.	Increased vibration
Percuss systematically over the lung area.	Resonant over lungs and dull over diaphragm	Asymmetrical sounds, dull over lungs, hyperresonance (pulmonary disease)

THE CHILD
An infant's chest is too small for reliable percussion.

THE ELDERLY
Hyperresonant sounds possible from hyperinflation of lung tissue.

ASSESSMENT TECHNIQUES: POSTERIOR THORAX (*CONTINUED*)

ASSESSMENT	NORMAL FINDINGS	DEVIATIONS FROM NORMAL
Percuss each side of posterior thorax for diaphragmatic excursion.	1¼ to 2¼ in excursion **NURSE ALERT:** The right side of the diaphragm is usually higher than the left.	Unequal excursion
Have patient take slow, deep breaths through mouth while you systematically auscultate the lungs. **THE CHILD** Auscultate a child first—other procedures may cause crying. **NURSE ALERT:** If the patient has a great deal of chest hair, moisten it to reduce interference.	Bronchial, vesicular, and bronchovesicular sounds **THE CHILD** A child may normally have coarser lung sounds.	Wheezing, coarse to fine crackles, rhonchi **NURSE ALERT:** Crackles may indicate congestive heart failure.

ASSESSMENT TECHNIQUES: ANTERIOR THORAX

ASSESSMENT	NORMAL FINDINGS	DEVIATIONS FROM NORMAL
Inspect anterior thoracic area.	Normal skin tone, symmetry of structures and inhalation	Abnormal skin tone, accessory muscle use, asymmetry, deformity, lifts, heaves, or thrusts, point of maximum impulse visible
	! **NURSE ALERT:** Children and men breathe with their diaphragm muscles, adult women breathe with their upper chest.	**!** **NURSE ALERT:** Children and very thin patients may normally have visible point of maximum impulse.
Palpate anterior thorax.	No tenderness or lesions	Lesions, lumps, pain, left and right symmetry
Inspect respiratory excursion.	Symmetrical expansion and contraction	Asymmetrical expansion and contraction

ASSESSMENT TECHNIQUES: ANTERIOR THORAX *(CONTINUED)*

ASSESSMENT	NORMAL FINDINGS	DEVIATIONS FROM NORMAL
Palpate as patient repeats "99" over and over. **THE CHILD** Unreliable in an infant.	Resonant lung fields, dullness over bony structures **THE ELDERLY** May have hyperresonant sounds.	Dullness over lung fields, abnormal sounds over bony structures
Perform a breast exam. **NURSE ALERT:** Have a patient with large, pendulous breasts lean forward.	Soft, symmetrical breasts, symmetrical nipples **THE PREGNANT PATIENT** Breasts are swollen, nipples dark, areola dark, may have purple streaks.	Asymmetry, abnormal hair growth, lesions, lumps, nodes, thickening; cracks, fissures, blisters, inflammation, pain, etc. **NURSE ALERT:** Culture any nipple discharge.
With patient at 45 degree angle, inspect jugular veins.	No pulsation	Distended, changes in bounding pulse

ASSESSMENT TECHNIQUES: ANTERIOR THORAX *(CONTINUED)*

ASSESSMENT	NORMAL FINDINGS	DEVIATIONS FROM NORMAL
Palpate precordium.	Point of maximum impulse at apical area	Shift in point of maximum impulse indicates abnormal changes in left ventricle
Auscultate for heart sounds.	S_1 and S_2, normal rhythm, pulse rate normal for age	Extra heart sounds, murmurs, rubs **THE CHILD** A child may have benign heart murmurs.

ASSESSMENT TECHNIQUES: ABDOMEN

ASSESSMENT	NORMAL FINDINGS	DEVIATIONS FROM NORMAL
Inspect abdomen.	Normal contour for body type and age, normal skin color	Asymmetry, bulges, visible growths, abnormal color, rash, visible peristaltic waves, hernia, lesions

ASSESSMENT TECHNIQUES: ABDOMEN *(CONTINUED)*

ASSESSMENT	NORMAL FINDINGS	DEVIATIONS FROM NORMAL
Systematically auscultate abdomen for up to 5 minutes in all four quadrants	Normal bowel sounds in all areas	Bruits, other abnormal sounds; hyperactive sounds in one area followed by absent sound

NURSE ALERT: Auscultate before percussion or palpation. If you perform either procedure first, you may generate abnormal sounds or rupture an aneurysm.

Percuss on left and right side from just below breast to midclavicular line.	Dull over liver, tympanic over abdomen	Abnormal sounds

NURSE ALERT: You may not feel the liver border if the patient has gas in the colon or congestion in the right lower lung.

ASSESSMENT TECHNIQUES: ABDOMEN (*CONTINUED*)

ASSESSMENT	NORMAL FINDINGS	DEVIATIONS FROM NORMAL
Systematically palpate abdomen, moving from upper to lower areas in each quadrant.	Soft, nontender symmetrical abdomen	Tenderness, masses, pain, bladder distention
NURSE ALERT: It helps a ticklish patient to place a hand over yours while you palpate.		**NURSE ALERT:** Examine any painful area last to prevent the patient from tensing to guard the area.
Palpate the liver.	Often nonpalpable; if edge palpable, smooth, nontender	Mushy, enlarged, lumps
Palpate the spleen.	Nonpalpable	Palpable (enlarged)
Palpate femoral groin pulse.	Symmetrical, strong	Asymmetrical, weak or absent
THE CHILD This is an important pulse point in children.		**NURSE ALERT:** Absent pulse with blue extremities is a clinical emergency.

ASSESSMENT TECHNIQUES: UPPER EXTREMITIES

ASSESSMENT	NORMAL FINDINGS	DEVIATIONS FROM NORMAL
Inspect the upper extremities. **THE CHILD** Skin turgor on the upper extremities and chest is important for identifying dehydration in infants and young children.	Normal, uniform skin color and texture, symmetrical muscle mass, good skin turgor **THE ELDERLY** Skin may be dry and thin with deficient turgor.	Abnormal color or texture, lesions, dryness, asymmetrical muscle mass, poor skin turgor
Have patient turn palms up and down with arms extended.	Steady hands, symmetrical movement	Tremors, pronator drift, unable to follow instructions
Have patient push forearms up and down against your hand.	Symmetrical strength and movement	Asymmetry when comparing left to right
Inspect and palpate all joints.	Normal range of motion	Stiffness, edema, enlarged joint, redness, pain with movement, limited range of motion

ASSESSMENT TECHNIQUES: UPPER EXTREMITIES (CONTINUED)

ASSESSMENT	NORMAL FINDINGS	DEVIATIONS FROM NORMAL
Palpate hands for temperature.	Warm, moist, symmetrical	Cool, clammy skin or warm, dry skin; asymmetry
Palpate brachial pulses.	Right and left equal	Decreased pulse strength, thready pulse, difference between right and left pulse
Inspect fingernails.	Color, shape, and condition normal, good capillary refill	Broken and cracked nails, pitting, clubbing, cyanosis, decreased capillary refill
Have patient squeeze two of your fingers with each fist.	Symmetry in hand strength	Asymmetry

ASSESSMENT TECHNIQUES: LOWER EXTREMITIES

ASSESSMENT	NORMAL FINDINGS	DEVIATIONS FROM NORMAL
Inspect lower extremities.	Even skin color and texture, symmetrical muscle mass, hair and nail growth	Abnormal color, lesions, dryness, hair loss, bruises, varicosity, edema, fungal toe nails, asymmetrical muscle mass

ASSESSMENT TECHNIQUES: LOWER EXTREMITIES *(CONTINUED)*

ASSESSMENT	NORMAL FINDINGS	DEVIATIONS FROM NORMAL
Palpate for pitting edema between knee and ankle and in foot.	No edema	Pitting edema present— grade according to scale
Palpate posterior tibial area and dorsalis pedis.	Symmetrical pulse, skin temperature	Asymmetrical, weak, or absent pulse; skin temperature decreases **NURSE ALERT:** If any pulse is abnormal, check the popliteal pulse.
Perform the straight leg test on each leg.	Normal movement **THE ELDERLY** May have difficulty with this test.	Pain with extension **NURSE ALERT:** Help a patient with difficulty extending by steadying leg.

ASSESSMENT TECHNIQUES: LOWER EXTREMITIES *(CONTINUED)*

ASSESSMENT	NORMAL FINDINGS	DEVIATIONS FROM NORMAL
Palpate hip with abduction and adduction.	No crepitus	Crepitus

THE CHILD
Use Ortolani's maneuver on an infant.

Have patient raise each thigh against your hand; push tibial area out against your hand; pull calf back against your hand.	Symmetrical strength	Weak or asymmetrical strength

THE CHILD
Test strength by having child hop on each leg.

𝒮UGGESTED READINGS

Anderson, F. D., and J. Malone. "Taking Blood Pressure." *Nursing94* 24 (November 1994): 34–39.

Flory, C. "Perfecting the Art of Skin Assessment." *RN* 55 (June 1992): 22–27.

Hartrick, G., and A. E. Lindsey. "Family Nursing Assessment: Meeting the Challenge of Health Promotion." *Journal of Advanced Nursing* 20 (July 1994): 85–91.

Jensen, L., and M. Allen. "Wellness—The Dialectic of Illness." *Image, Journal of Nursing Scholarship* 2 (Fall 1993): 220–224.

SECTION II. CARDIOVASCULAR ASSESSMENT

$\mathscr{C}$hapter 4. Anatomy and Physiology

▽   ▽   ▽   ▽   ▽   ▽   ▽

$\mathscr{I}$NTRODUCTION

SEE TEXT PAGES

This chapter provides an overview of the heart—what it's made of and how it works. Illustrations are provided throughout to support the text.

$\mathscr{A}$NATOMY

Cardiac Muscle

Unlike the skeletal muscle, cardiac muscle has more mitochondria. It is also able to produce more adenosine triphosphate. Intercalated discs connect the muscle fibers in a lattice structure known as the functional syncytium. All fibers in the syncytium contract when one fiber contracts.

Cardiac muscle cells have the following special properties:
- Excitability—the ability to depolarize when stimulated.
- Conductivity—the ability to carry electrical impulses to other cells. This allows the heart to achieve full depolarization.
- Refractoriness—temporarily inhibits depolarized cells from reacting to a stimulus.
- Automaticity—the cardiac pacemaker cells in the sinoatrial (SA) and atrioventricular (AV) nodes can reach threshold and depolarize without external stimuli.
- Contractility—muscle cell contracts as a unit, once depolarized.

The Heart's Structures

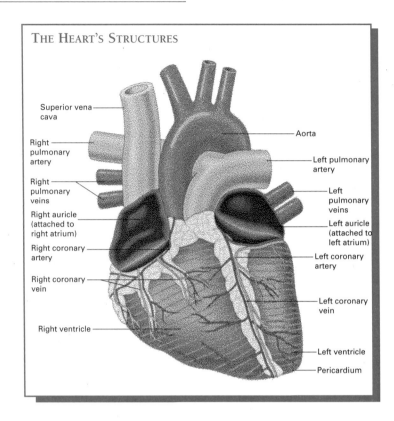

- Superior vena cava
- Right pulmonary artery
- Right pulmonary veins
- Right auricle (attached to right atrium)
- Right coronary artery
- Right coronary vein
- Right ventricle
- Aorta
- Left pulmonary artery
- Left pulmonary veins
- Left auricle (attached to left atrium)
- Left coronary artery
- Left coronary vein
- Left ventricle
- Pericardium

THE CARDIAC WALL

STRUCTURE	DESCRIPTION
Pericardium	Membranous sac around heart and roots of great vessels that protects the heart from friction. The outermost layer is the fibrous pericardium. The serous pericardium has two layers, the parietal layer and the visceral layer that cover and protect the heart.
Epicardium	The visceral layer of the serous pericardium. It covers the heart and the great vessels.
Myocardium	Heart muscle composed of cardiac muscle cells

THE CARDIAC WALL (CONTINUED)

STRUCTURE	DESCRIPTION
Endocardium	Heart's inner membrane that provides lining for the chambers
Papillary muscles	Extend from the ventricular myocardial surfaces to the chordae tendineae
Chordae tendineae	Tendons between the papillary muscles and the tricuspid and mitral valves that prevent the valves from everting into the atria during systole

THE HEART'S CHAMBERS

Chambers consist of the atria and ventricles. The atria are the heart's receiving chambers. During early diastole, 70% of the blood moves passively from the atria to the ventricles. The rest of the blood for ventricular stroke volume is actively added by atrial contraction (or atrial kick). The ventricles are the main pumps of the heart.

CHAMBER	FUNCTION
Right atrium (RA)	To receive systemic venous blood from the superior vena cava, inferior vena cava, and coronary sinus
Left atrium (LA)	To receive oxygenated blood from the lungs through the four pulmonary veins
Right ventricle (RV)	A low-pressure system that forces deoxygenated blood through pulmonary artery into pulmonary circulatory system
Left ventricle (LV)	Heart's primary pump; a high-pressure system that forces blood into systemic circulation throughout the aorta during systole

Valves

There are two types of cardiac valves—atrioventricular and semilunar. The atrioventricular valves are the mitral valve between the LA and LV and the tricuspid valve between the RA and RV. The valves allow blood to flow in one direction from the atria to the ventricles during diastole. Their function is to prevent backflow into the atria during systole. The closing of the atrioventricular valves causes the first heart sound, S_1. The first heart sound has two components, mitral (M_1) and tricuspid (T_1) but are normally heard as one sound—S_1.

The semilunar valves are the pulmonary valve between the RV and pulmonary artery and the aortic valve between the LV and aorta. These valves allow blood to flow from the outflow tract during systole. Their most important function is to prevent backflow into the ventricle during diastole. The closing of the semilunar valves causes the second heart sound, S_2. The second heart sound also has two components, aortic (A_2) and pulmonic (P_2) valve closures and are also normally heard as one sound—S_2.

Systemic Circulation and Vessels

The circulatory system is a vast network. Its center is the heart, which continuously circulates approximately 10 pints of blood in an adult. That blood is moved to and from every living cell.

The systemic circulation supplies tissues with blood and nutrients. The vessels also remove waste products. Blood flow is controlled by means of three mechanisms: local, nervous, and humoral. Vessel diameter, blood viscosity, and vessel wall elasticity determine resistance to flow.

CORONARY ARTERY BLOOD FLOW DISTRIBUTION

The arteries that come from the base of the aorta, providing blood to the myocardium and the electrical conduction system, compose the coronary vasculature.

COMPONENT	FUNCTION
Right coronary artery (RCA)	Provides blood to the SA node in 55% of patients, to the AV node in 90% of patients, to the RA and RV heart muscle, and to the inferioposterior LV wall In 80% of patients there is also a branch, the posterior descending artery, that provides blood to the RV and the LV inferior wall as well as to the posterior interventricular septum. The RCA is called "dominant" in such patients.
Left main coronary artery (LMCA)	Supplies blood to left anterior descending artery and circumflex
Left anterior descending artery (LAD)	Provides blood to anterior of interventricular septum, LV anterior wall, right bundle branch, left bundle branch anterosuperior division
Circumflex	Provides blood to AV node in 10% of patients, SA node in 45% of patients, LV lateral posterior surface
Veins: great cardiac, small cardiac, thebesian	Returns deoxygenated blood to heart

𝒯HE VASCULAR SYSTEM

The vascular system is composed of the following:
- Arteries. A high-pressure circuit consisting of strong elastic vessels that carry blood from the heart through the capillary beds to the body. Arteries expand during systole and contract during diastole.

- Arterioles. Smooth muscle that constricts when stimulated by the autonomic nervous system. They control blood distribution to capillary beds by dilating in reaction to decreased adrenergic discharge. These vessels control vascular resistance and arterial pressure.
- Capillary system. Provides exchange of oxygen and carbon dioxide nutrients between vessels and tissues, and controls fluid volume transfer between plasma and interstitium.
- Venous system. Warehouse for 65% of total blood volume; composed of veins and venules, which accept blood from the capillaries and conduct it back to the heart. The venous pump consists of veins surrounded by skeletal muscles. Muscle contraction moves the blood to the heart. Valves prevent backflow.

Factors Affecting LV Function

Preload is the tension of the muscle caused by blood volume at the end of diastole.

Afterload is the tension of the muscle caused by the resistance to flow into the systemic circulation across the aortic valve at the onset of systole.

Contractility is the strength of myocardial muscle work. It is affected by preload, afterload, and the condition of the heart muscle.

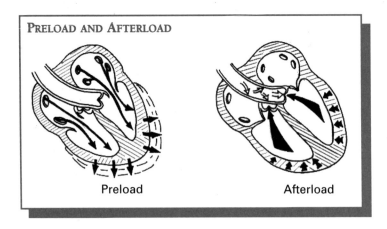

PRELOAD AND AFTERLOAD

Preload   Afterload

Arterial Pressure

Along with mechanisms in the peripheral blood vessels, the following factors control arterial pressure:

- The hormone renin, which is secreted by the kidneys and converts angiotensin I to angiotensin II, causing vasoconstriction
- Capillary fluid shift
- Local control mechanisms
- Fluid retention or excretion (renal)
- Miscellaneous factors, including cardiac output, heart rate, systemic vascular resistance, arterial elasticity, blood volume, blood viscosity, age, body surface area, exercise, emotional state, and sodium retention.

Other Considerations

- Pulse pressure—the numerical difference between systolic and diastolic pressure measured in millimeters of mercury (mm Hg).
- Mean arterial pressure, or the average aortic and arterial pressures during a cardiac cycle, is a function of cardiac output and vascular resistance.

THE CONDUCTION SYSTEM

The conduction system consists of the following:

- Sinoatrial (SA) node—heart's pacemaker
- Internodal atrial pathways—composed of the anterior, middle, and posterior tracts, these pathways carry the SA node impulse throughout the RA musculature to the AV node.
- Bachman's bundle—carries SA node impulse to LA
- AV node—delays the impulse between the atria and ventricles so that ventricular filling can be completed
- Bundle of His—carries impulse from AV node to bundle branches.
- Bundle branch system—consists of right and left bundle branch coming from the bundle of His. The right bundle, which continues from the bundle of His, carries the impulse throughout the right side of the interventricular septum to the RV myocardium. The left bundle branch divides into the left posterior fascicle and the left anterior fascicle. The impulse is transmitted to anterior, posterior, septal, and inferior endocardium.
- Purkinje system—continues from the distal portion of bundle branches and carries the impulse into ventricular subendocardial layers. It depolarizes from the endocardium to the epicardium, with ventricular contraction and blood ejection from ventricles after depolarization.

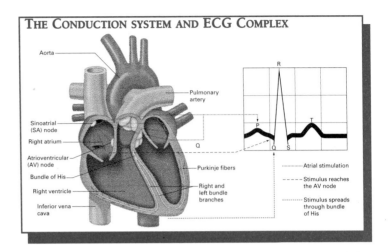

THE CONDUCTION SYSTEM AND ECG COMPLEX

Electrical Activity and the Cardiac Cycle

The electrical activity of the heart initiates the following:

- Atrial depolarization results in a P wave. Atrial pressure exceeds ventricular pressure due to venous return during atrial diastole. AV valves open (mitral and tricuspid).
- The higher pressure in the atria passively pushes blood into the ventricle (ventricular diastole).
- Atrial systole occurs. Active contraction of the atria contributes 20% to 30% of the cardiac output to the ventricles.
- The ventricles depolarize. The QRS complex appears on ECG.
- The AV valves close in response to the rise in pressure in the ventricle. S_1 is heard. Ventricular systole starts.
- Early systole (phase I of ventricular contraction) occurs when pressure increases, but there is no blood movement from the ventricles.
- LV pressure becomes greater than aortic pressure and the aortic valve opens.
- Blood is ejected into the aorta. This is the main systolic event.
- As LV blood outflow decreases and ventricular ejection ends, LV pressure drops below aortic pressure.
- Backflow of blood occurs from the aorta to the LV, forcing the aortic and pulmonary valves to close, producing S_2. Ventricular systole is completed.
- The ventricles repolarize.
- Once the aortic valve closes, LV pressure quickly drops. No blood flows into the ventricle.

- Now the ventricular pressure is lower than atrial pressure, and the AV valves open, beginning the next ventricular diastolic event.

ASSESSING AUTONOMIC REGULATION

The autonomic nervous system, chemoreceptors, stretch receptors, and the respiratory reflex provide autonomic regulation of the heart. The following table describes the function of each component responsible for autonomic regulation.

COMPONENT	FUNCTION
Autonomic nervous system	Sympathetic stimulation releases norepinephrine to • trigger vasoconstriction of the arteries • increase heart rate by increasing SA nodal discharge • increase myocardial contraction • speedup AV conduction Parasympathetic stimulation releases acetylcholine to • lower heart rate by lowering SA nodal discharge • slow AV conduction
Chemoreceptors	Change heart and respiratory rate in response to changes in Pao_2, $Paco_2$, and pH
Stretch receptors	Located in aortic arch, carotid sinus, vena cava, pulmonary artery, and atria; react to changes in pressure and volume
Respiratory reflex	Inspiration • decreases intrathoracic pressure, which increases venous return • stimulates lung and thorax stretch receptors • decreases vagal tone, which increases heart rate and blood volume

Chapter 5. Subjective Data Collection

▽   ▽   ▽   ▽   ▽   ▽   ▽

INTRODUCTION

SEE TEXT PAGES

When collecting a cardiovascular health history, you will want to gather any information about your patient's risk factors, including lifestyle and any symptoms of heart disease.

SUPPORTING ASSESSMENT DATA

If your assessment findings are similar to those listed here, they may suggest cardiovascular disease.

▼
▼
▼
▼
▼
▼
▼
▼
▼

▲ Risk Factors:

The following factors increase your patient's risk of heart disease:
• Blood relative with cardiac disease before age 55
• Male
• Post menopausal female
• African-American women of any age; African-American, Puerto Rican, Cuban, and Mexican men are at higher risk of hypertension
• Native American over age 35 (twice the risk)
• African-American man (twice the risk for stroke)
• Over age 60 (three times the risk)
• Cigarette smoking
• Hyperlipidemia (elevated lipid count)
• Diabetes mellitus
• Obesity
• Sedentary lifestyle
• Stress
• High-fat diet
• LV hypertrophy
• Use of oral contraceptives
• Gout

▲ Physical Findings:

The following symptoms indicate a patient with or at risk for cardiovascular disease:
• Chest pain
• Dyspnea
• Orthopnea
• Cough
• Fatigue
• Cyanosis
• Pallor

- Edema
- Intermittent claudication (peripheral vascular disease)
- Clubbing
- Arrhythmias
- Nocturia

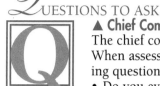

UESTIONS TO ASK

▲ Chief Complaint:

The chief complaint should be in the patient's own words. When assessing the patient's chief complaint, ask the following questions.
- Do you ever have chest pressure, heaviness, or pain?
- Do you ever feel fatigued? Tired?
- Have you ever noticed swelling in your ankles, feet, or hands? How long have you had this?
- Are you ever confused?
- Has your skin ever appeared bluish?
- Have you ever had palpitations?
- Have you ever been short of breath?
- Are you ever dizzy or have you ever fainted?
- Have these problems adversely affected your life?

▲ Health History of Present Illness:

When assessing the patient's present illness, ask the following questions:
- When did your symptoms start?
- Does your heart pound after exertion?
- When changing position, do you ever feel dizzy?
- Does your heart ever pound, race, or feel as though it is skipping beats?
- Do you tire easily? With what activity? Does rest help?
- Are there any ulcers or sores on your legs? How are they healing? Is there any change in feeling?
- Are you rested when you awaken? Tired during the day? Do you take naps?
- Do you have to get up during the night to urinate?
- During the night do you become short of breath?
- Cough? When and how often?
- Do you have to prop yourself up in bed because you are short of breath?
- Does the weather affect your symptoms? What kind of weather and how?
- Do you have leg pain with walking?
- Have you felt fatigued recently?

▲ Past Medical History:

When assessing past medical history, ask the following quetions:
- Have you ever had chest pain?
- Do you have high blood pressure?

- Are you anemic?
- Do you have allergies?
- Do you ever find yourself short of breath? If so, do you cough?
- Have you had any recent dental work or surgery? Cystoscopy or other similar procedure? When?
- Have you ever had high cholesterol or diabetes? When were you diagnosed? What treatment do you follow? Has it affected your lifestyle? How?
- Have you ever had a positive stress test?
- Have you ever had an EPS (electrophysiologic) study?
- Do you have a congenital heart problem? When was it diagnosed? How was it treated?
- Have you had rheumatic fever? When? Any heart problems from it?
- Do you have a heart murmur? When was it diagnosed? Any treatment?
- Are you enrolled in any experimental drug protocols?
- Have you ever had cardiac catheterization, cardiac artery bypass surgery, valve replacement, carotid endarterectomy, femoral bypass, or abdominal aneurysm repair?

▲ Medication History:

When assessing the patient's medication history, ask the following questions:
- What heart medications do you take?
- What over-the-counter medications do you take?
- Do you take any prescription medications?

▲ Family History:

When assessing family history, ask the following questions:
- Do you have a family history of heart disease? What family member? At what age?
- Do you have any relatives who died suddenly for no apparent cause?
- Do you have any family history of high blood pressure, obesity, high cholesterol, or diabetes mellitus? Who? Onset at what age? Treatment?

▲ Social History:

When assessing the patient's social history, ask the following questions:
- Do you drink alcohol? What type? How often? How many drinks over how long?
- Do you smoke? If yes, how many packs per day? For how many years?
- When you feel stressed, what is the cause? Any physical symptoms?
- What have you eaten in the past 3 days?

- Do you use drugs like cocaine? How often?
- What is the layout of your living space? Are there any steps to climb?
- Do you exercise regularly? What type of exercise? How often and for how long?
- Have you had any change in exercise level over the past 6 months? In the past year? Five years? Why?
- Have you had any change in sexual activity? What kind of change? How do you feel about it?

AMBULATORY CARE

Ask ambulatory patients the following questions:
- Do you wear a medical alert identification?
- If you have a pacemaker or automatic implanted cardiovascular defibrillator, do you carry a card listing its settings?

TYPES OF CHEST PAIN

Chest pain is not always caused by heart problems. The following table provides a description of the type of chest pain experienced with different types of disease.

DISEASE STATE	PAIN
Angina **NURSE ALERT:** Women may have atypical anginal symptoms.	Patient describes as crushing, squeezing, heavy, tight, aching, like indigestion that begins either suddenly or gradually and subsides in 5 to 10 minutes. Often relieved by rest or sublingual nitroglycerin.
Mitral valve prolapse	Patient may describe pressure or sharp stabbing pain. May have dyspnea if regurgitation is present.
Myocardial infarction	Patient describes as crushing, squeezing, heavy, tight, aching, like indigestion that begins either suddenly or gradually and is constant. Is not relieved by rest.
Pericarditis	Patient describes as sharp or stabbing, with sudden onset and constant duration.
Postmyocardial syndrome (Dressler's syndrome)	Patient describes as sharp or stabbing, with sudden onset (1 week to 12 months after infarction) and of constant duration.

TYPES OF CHEST PAIN (CONTINUED)

DISEASE STATE	PAIN
Dissecting aortic aneurysm	Patient feels as though chest is being ripped or torn; or complains of throbbing heart.
Pulmonary artery hypertension	Patient describes as crushing or gripping with sudden onset, usually at night. May be intermittent or constant.
Pulmonary embolism	Patient describes as sharp, stabbing, gripping, worse with deep breath. May have difficulty breathing. Sudden onset and short duration.
Pneumonia	Patient describes as burning, sharp, stabbing, or tearing, with sudden or gradual onset, lasting from days to weeks.
Rib fracture	Patient describes as sore, stabbing, being stuck, pain with movement, onset with or after meal, lasting from 10 minutes to 1 hour, or may last for weeks.
Esophageal reflux	Patient describes as heartburn, dull, burning, squeezing with onset with or after meal, lasting from 10 minutes to 1 hour.
Esophageal spasm	Patient describes as recurrent dull, burning, crushing, gripping, squeezing, pressure with sudden onset, lasting from seconds to minutes.

!

NURSE ALERT:
Symptoms may be relieved with sublingual nitroglycerin due to relaxation effects on esophageal smooth muscle.

Hiatal hernia	Patient describes as dull, full, or heavy with onset 1 to 4 hours after eating.
Cholecystitis	Patient describes as radiating heartburn, indigestion, epigastric heaviness, with onset 30 to 60 minutes after eating.

Ꮸhapter 6. Objective Data Collection

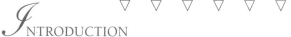

ᏋNTRODUCTION

SEE TEXT PAGES

This chapter is a guide to the physical assessment of the cardiac patient.

ᏇOOLS OF THE TRADE

In performing a physical assessment you need the following tools:
- Drapes
- ECG calipers
- Gown
- Ruler
- Scale
- Sphygmomanometer
- Stethoscope

INSPECTION FOR CARDIAC ASSESSMENT

AREA	METHOD	LOOK FOR
General	Observation	• General appearance of health or illness • Skin color, temperature, moisture, turgor, angiomas, ulcers, petechiae
Thorax	Observation	• Heaves or thrusts over precordial area • Chest symmetry and contour • Respiration • Pulses • Any visible point of maximal impulse

INSPECTION FOR CARDIAC ASSESSMENT (*CONTINUED*)

AREA	METHOD	LOOK FOR
Neck veins	• Place patient at 45 degree angle. • Illuminate vessels. • Sternal angle is 5 cm above the atrium. • Take measurement (cm) from sternal angle to top of distended vein. • Measurement plus 5 cm is the central venous pressure.	• Distention • Pulsation • Central venous pressure
Extremities	Check both sides; should be symmetrical	• Nail bed color, clubbing, refill • Edema • Color • Temperature • Hair distribution • Peripheral pulses • Blood pressure • Ulceration

INTERPRETING INSPECTION FINDINGS

AREA	NORMAL FINDINGS	DEVIATIONS FROM NORMAL
Jugular veins • Have patient lie down without a pillow. • Elevate torso 45 degrees. • Shine a penlight tangential to neck to show pulsations and shadows. • Use two rulers to measure the highest visible point of the internal jugular vein on each side.	No distention, pulsation, venous pressure ≥ 2 cm	• Unilateral distention (kinking or aneurysm) • Fully distended (elevated central venous pressure)

INTERPRETING INSPECTION FINDINGS (CONTINUED)

AREA	NORMAL FINDINGS	DEVIATIONS FROM NORMAL
Anterior chest	Apical impulse may or may not be visible (more likely to see in a child or thin patient)	Heave or lift at sternal border or apex (ventricular hypertrophy)

PALPATION FOR CARDIAC ASSESSMENT

AREA	TECHNIQUE	LOOK FOR
Arteries, including carotid, brachial, radial, femoral, popliteal, dorsalis pedis, posterior tibialis	On scale of 0 to 3: • 0 = no pulse • 1 = thready, very weak • 2 = normal • 3 = bounding, hard	0, 1, or 3 as abnormals
	On palpation, surging pulse preceding an abrupt absence of force	Pulsus magnus—3+ bounding pulse
	On palpation, regular pulse, which alternates in force	Pulsus alternans—alternate beat weaker than preceding beat
	On palpation, pulse with close attention to quality during inspiration. Correlate with blood pressure readings.	Pulsus paradoxus—>10 mm Hg drop in arterial systolic pressure during inspiration

PALPATION FOR CARDIAC ASSESSMENT *(CONTINUED)*

AREA	TECHNIQUE	LOOK FOR
Arteries *(continued)*	Palpate pulse upstroke with close attention to upstroke and downstroke. **NURSE ALERT** Palpate pulse carefully during periods of arrhythmia to determine perfusion, especially of premature beats.	Pulsus biferiens— double beat during systole
Precordium	Palpate the sternoclavicular, aortic, pulmonic, epigastric, and apical areas. The point of maximal impulse is located at the fifth intercostal space, midclavicular line; pulsations should be palpated strongest here.	Abnormal point of maximum impulse • Lateral displacement of apical impulse >7–9 cm from left sternal border • Medial displacement of apical impulse • Hard, enduring apical impulse • Vibrations, pulsations in any area

INTERPRETING PALPATION FINDINGS

AREA	TECHNIQUE	LOOK FOR
Anterior chest	No pulsations Palpate the following areas: • Along angle of Louis (sternal angle) • Adjacent second ribs	Pulsations

INTERPRETING PALPATION FINDINGS *(CONTINUED)*

AREA	TECHNIQUE	LOOK FOR
Apical impulse (point of maximal impulse)	• Occupies only fourth or fifth interspace medial to the midclavicular line • 1 x 2 cm in size • Short, gentle tap • Occurs in first half of systole	• Displaced down and to left; occupies more than one space (LV dilation) • Location correct, but elevated force and duration (LV of systole hypertrophy) • Not palpable (pulmonary emphysema; obesity; very muscular, large breasts)
Carotid artery Be gentle and palpate one artery at a time. NURSE ALERT: *Do not* palpate both arteries simultaneously. You may inadvertently reduce or cut off blood supply to the brain or cause vagal bradycardia.	Smooth contour, upstroke more rapid than downstroke, 2+ strength, symmetrical	• Diminished pulse with decreased stroke volume (narrowing of artery) • Increased pulse with hyperkinesis • Change in regularity of pulse as patient breathes in (sinus dysrhythmia) • Change in regularity of pulse as patient exhales • Asymmetry
Precordium • Use the palmar aspect to gently palpate. • Palpate the apex. • Palpate the left sternal border. • Palpate the base.	No pulsations	• Pulsations—note timing • Thrill (like a purring cat) indicates a murmur

INTERPRETING PALPATION FINDINGS (CONTINUED)

AREA	TECHNIQUE	LOOK FOR
Lower extremities	Palpate for edema	Pitting edema

INTERPRETING AUSCULTATION FINDINGS

AUSCULTATION TECHNIQUE	NORMAL FINDINGS	DEVIATIONS FROM NORMAL
Carotid artery **THE ELDERLY:** Perform this procedure on patients who are past middle age or who show signs of cardiovascular problems. **NURSE ALERT:** Have the patient hold his or her breath.	No turbulence, pulse synchronous with apical pulse	• Bruit—indicative of turbulence, usually caused by athero-sclerotic narrowing in arteries • Murmur—similar to a bruit but radiates from the aortic valve in the heart
Heart sounds (S_1 and S_2) When auscultating heart sounds, count the heart rate (S_1 and S_2 as one heartbeat) and note the time between S_1 and S_2 and then between S_2 and S_1 (heart rhythm).	• S_1 at onset of ventricular systole—clearest at apex • S_2 at end of ventricular systole—clearest at base	• Fixed splitting of S_2 that does not disappear when patient exhales 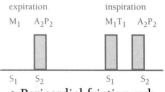 • Pericardial friction rub

INTERPRETING AUSCULTATION FINDINGS *(CONTINUED)*

AUSCULTATION TECHNIQUE	NORMAL FINDINGS	DEVIATIONS FROM NORMAL
Heart sounds (S_1 and S_2) *(continued)*	• Diastolic period between S_2 and S_1 is longer than the systolic period between S_1 and S_2	• Paradoxical splitting of S_2 that disappears when patient inhales 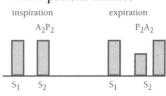
	• Split S_1 (M_1T_1) Common—physiologic split S_1—hear mitral valve (M_1) closing before tricuspid valve (T_1). Loudest at apex.	• Diminished S_1 • Accentuated S_1 • Diminished S_2 • Accentuated S_2 • Premature beat • Random, rapid beat • Irregular heart rhythm
	  NURSE ALERT: Do not confuse this with an atrial gallop before M_1. This is abnomal. • Split S_2 (A_2P_2) • Normal physiologic splitting of S_2-P_2 delayed on inspiration due to pulmonary valve (P_2) closing after aortic valve (A_2)	 **NURSE ALERT:** Examine the patient for a pulse deficit. If you have one examiner, you can do this by listening to the apical pulse while palpating the radial pulse. If you have two examiners, you can both compare the two rates at the same time. Report pulse deficit to a physician as soon as possible.

INTERPRETING AUSCULTATION FINDINGS (*CONTINUED*)

AUSCULTATION TECHNIQUE	NORMAL FINDINGS	DEVIATIONS FROM NORMAL
Heart sounds (S_3) Third heart sound auscultated during diastole. S_3 occurs at the apex or lower left sternal border. **NURSE ALERT:** Auscultate lungs for crackles if a new S_3 is heard.	Not a normal finding **THE CHILD** Children and young adults may normally have physiologic S_3. S_3 is abnormal in the older adult or in disease states.	Ventricular gallop (pathologic S_3) in adults sounds like "KEN-TUC-KEY" low-pitched 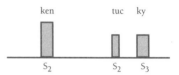 **NURSE ALERT:** Be careful not to confuse this with a split S_2. The split occurs at the base. S_3 does not vary as patient breathes. The split varies. S_3 is low-pitched and the split has a constant pitch.
Heart sounds (S_4) Fourth heart sound auscultated during diastole. S_4 heard at apex or lower left sternal border.	Not a normal finding	Atrial gallop (pathologic S_4) in adults sounds like "TEN-NES-SEE" 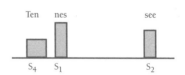 **THE ELDERLY:** S_4 may normally occur in an older patient.

INTERPRETING AUSCULTATION FINDINGS *(CONTINUED)*

AUSCULTATION TECHNIQUE	NORMAL FINDINGS	DEVIATIONS FROM NORMAL
Heart sounds (S_3 and S_4)	Not a normal finding	• Summation gallop (S_3 and S_4 simultaneously)

slower heart rates

S_1 S_2 S_3 S_4 S_1

heart rates over 100/min

S_1 S_2 S_{3+4}

Abnormal Heart Sounds

The table on the next page describes the murmurs/sounds caused by various cardiac conditions. Note a murmur in terms of its timing (systole or diastole), its loudness, and whether the sound radiates.

Loudness is graded as follows:
• Grade 1—Very soft, hard to hear
• Grade 2—Faint, but can be heard clearly
• Grade 3—Somewhat loud
• Grade 4—Loud and accompanied by a chest wall thrill that you can palpate
• Grade 5—Very loud; can be heard when you partially lift stethoscope away from chest wall
• Grade 6—Extremely loud; can be heard when you hold stethoscope just above chest wall

MURMURS AND SOUNDS CAUSED BY CARDIAC CONDITIONS

ASSESSMENT AREA	NORMAL FINDINGS	DEVIATIONS FROM NORMAL
Systolic murmurs	No murmur at systole **THE CHILD:** Children and adolescents may have systolic murmurs that are not pathological. However, you should investigate any murmur that you hear.	Systolic murmur: • Mitral insufficiency (see Chapter 14, "Mitral Insufficiency"): pansystolic, blowing, high-pitched • Tricuspid insufficiency: pansystolic, blowing, high-pitched • Hypertrophic cardiomyopathy: crescendo-decrescendo, ejection murmur (peaks in intensity) Crescendo-decrescendo 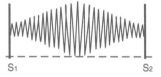 Ejection murmur 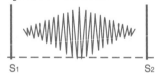 • Interventricular defect: pansystolic Pansystolic 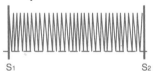

MURMURS AND SOUNDS *(CONTINUED)*

ASSESSMENT AREA	NORMAL FINDINGS	DEVIATIONS FROM NORMAL
Diastolic murmurs	No murmur at diastole	Diastolic murmur: • Mitral stenosis: (see Chapter 13, "Mitral Stenosis") mid-diastolic or prediastolic rumble, often faint. No increase in intensity with inspiration. • Tricuspid stenosis: Left sternum protodiastolic, decrescendo, increases with inspiration

Protodiastolic

S₁   S₂   S₁

Decrescendo

S₁   S₂

• Aortic insufficiency (see Chapter 16, "Aortic Insufficiency"):
• Pulmonary insufficiency
• Patent ductus arteriosus

MURMURS AND SOUNDS (CONTINUED)

ASSESSMENT AREA	NORMAL FINDINGS	DEVIATIONS FROM NORMAL
Lungs Have patient breathe deeply through mouth. Lungs should be symmetrical in sound.	• Vesicular sounds over anterior, lateral, and posterior chest • Bronchial sounds over the trachea • Bronchovesicular sounds over large bronchi near sternum, between scapulae and apex on right upper lobe **NURSE ALERT:** Avoid extraneous sounds that are produced by moving the stethoscope or your hands during auscultation.	• Absent or diminished sounds, indicative of obstruction, pulmonary disease, weak muscles, splinting due to pain • Bronchial sounds over bases instead of trachea indicate consolidation • Bronchovesicular over lungs rather than large bronchi indicate consolidation • Crackles when patient inhales that do not clear with coughing; can be fine or coarse **NURSE ALERT:** Crackles at the lung base may be an early indicator of congestive heart failure. Check weight and peripheral edema. May require follow-up chest X-rays.

MURMURS AND SOUNDS (CONTINUED)

ASSESSMENT AREA	NORMAL FINDINGS	DEVIATIONS FROM NORMAL
Lungs (continued)		• Wheezing—check if with coughing • Rhonchi or gurgles heard during respiratory cycle in central airway • Stridor when the patient inhales, located in trachea • Grunting when the patient exhales • Pleural friction rub in the lateral lung field during respiratory cycle • Mediastinal crunch heard when air is in pericardium and/or mediastinum
Blood pressure Take the blood pressures while the patient sits, lies down, and stands.	Blood pressure less than 140/90 THE PREGNANT PATIENT Blood pressure is normally low. .	Blood pressure greater than 140/90 THE PREGNANT PATIENT A sustained elevation of 30 mm Hg systolic or 15 mm Hg diastolic indicates pregnancy-induced hypertension.

MURMURS AND SOUNDS *(CONTINUED)*

ASSESSMENT AREA	NORMAL FINDINGS	DEVIATIONS FROM NORMAL
Blood pressure *(continued)*	**THE ELDERLY** Slightly elevated systolic blood pressure can be normal with aging. Elderly patients may experience a sudden drop in blood pressure when standing up.	

ABNORMAL HEART SOUNDS

SOUND	FEATURES	INDICATIVE OF
Accentuated S_1	Beginning of systole	Fever, mitral stenosis
Accentuated S_2	End of systole	Hypertension
Diminished S_1	Beginning of systole	Obesity, emphysema, pericardial fluid, heart block, mitral insufficiency
Diminished/absent S_2	End of systole	Aortic stenosis, pulmonary stenosis, pericardial effusion
Fixed splitting of S_2	End of systole; no respiratory variation	Right bundle branch block, atrial septal defect, pulmonary stenosis, mitral insufficiency, pulmonary hypertension, sickle cell anemia
Paradoxical splitting of S_2	Most intense at second intercostal space; begins with ventricular systole; loudest at apex due to delayed aortic valve closure	Left bundle branch block, severe aortic stenosis, patent ductus arteriosus
Ventricular S_3 gallop	Early diastole, caused by resistance to ventricular filling from volume overload or decreased compliance. Heard at apex, low-pitched; with bell of stethoscope sounds like "KEN-TUC-KY"	Mitral insufficiency, tricuspid insufficiency, ischemia, congestive heart failure, left-to-right shunts **THE CHILD** Normal in children and adolescents.

ABNORMAL HEART SOUNDS (CONTINUED)

SOUND	FEATURES	INDICATIVE OF
Atrial S_4 gallop	Late diastole; occurs with atrial contraction when diastolic pressure is increased, usually due to RV or LV overload	LV, LA hypertrophy, myocardial infarction, congestive heart failure pulmonary stenosis, coronary artery disease, aortic stenosis
	Right-sided S_4 louder on inspiration; left-sided S_4 louder on expiration; sounds like "TEN-NES-SEE"	
Summation gallop (S_3 and S_4 together) **!** **NURSE ALERT:** Auscultate lungs for crackles.	Mid-diastole caused by shortened diastolic filling time; sounds like galloping hooves	Advanced congestive heart failure, tachycardia
Click	High-pitched, short extra sound	Pulmonary systolic ejection—indicates pulmonary stenosis
Pericardial friction rub	Squeaky, rubbing sound-grating at left sternal border; muffled, high-pitched, transient	Pericarditis

LABORATORY TESTS

Various tests are used to assess heart structure and functions. Each of the following chapters in this book lists pertinent tests related to specific disorders. To complete your cardiac assessment, consult the appropriate chapter.

Some of the most common tests are echocardiography, exercise stress testing with thallium or Cardiolite, 24-hour Holter monitoring, and multiple-gaited acquisition scan.

THE ECG

The ECG is one of the most important evaluations of the heart. The following provides a description of the information you are likely to see on an ECG strip.

- The isoelectric line is a straight line on the ECG with no electrical activity.
- The P wave (first positive deflection) represents depolarization of the atria.
- The PR interval reflects atrial depolarization and conduction through the AV node. The PR interval ranges from 0.12 to 0.20 seconds, measured from the beginning of the P wave to the start of the QRS complex.
- The QRS complex reflects total ventricular depolarization. Normal ranges from 0.06 to 0.12 seconds.
  - Q wave (first negative deflection)
  - R wave (first positive deflection)
  - S wave (negative deflection after R wave)
- ST segment reflects the beginning of ventricular repolarization measured from the end of QRS to the beginning of T wave.
- T wave (positive deflection) represents ventricular repolarization.
- QT interval reflects the sum of ventricular depolarization and repolarization measured from Q wave to the end of the T wave. Normal timing varies with heart rate.

Variations on the ECG are essential for arrhythmia detection and provide information on electrolyte imbalances, ischemia, and cardiac disease states. The 12-lead ECG assists in diagnosis of myocardial infarction and conduction disturbances.

UGGESTED READINGS

Clark, J. R. "Listen Closely: Assessing Heart Sounds." *Journal of Emergency Medical Services* 18 (1993): 46–67.

Dillon, P. "Self-Test: Reviewing Cardiac Assessment Skills." *Nursing93* 23 (1993): 76-78.

Fabius, D. B. "Understanding Heart Sounds: Solving the Mystery of Heart Murmurs." *Nursing94* 24 (1994): 39–44.

Fabius, D. B. "Understanding Heart Sounds: Uncovering the Secrets of Snaps, Rubs, and Clicks." *Nursing94* 24 (1994): 45–50.

Green, E. "Solving the Puzzle of Chest Pain." *AJN* 92 (1992): 32–37.

Hollerbach, A. D. "Accuracy of Radial Pulse Assessment by Length of Counting Interval." *Heart & Lung* 19 (1990).

McGovern, M., and J. K. Kuhn. "Cardiac Assessment of the Elderly Client." *Journal of Gerontological Nursing* 18 (1992): 40–44.

Yacone-Morton, L. A. "Perfecting the Art of Cardiac Assessment." *RN* 54 (1991): 28–35.

Chapter 7. Coronary Artery Disease

▽ ▽ ▽ ▽ ▽ ▽ ▽

INTRODUCTION

SEE TEXT PAGES

Coronary artery disease (CAD) is one of the leading causes of death of men and women in the United States.

SUPPORTING ASSESSMENT DATA

If your assessment findings are similar to those listed here, they may suggest CAD.

▼
▼
▼
▼
▼
▼
▼
▼
▼

▲ Health History:

The following factors increase the risk of CAD:
• Close blood relative with the disease
• Increased risk after age 40
• Men (white men are at a greater risk than nonwhite men)
• Hypertension
• Post menopausal women (same incidence as men; nonwhite women have a greater risk than white women)
• Diabetes mellitus
• Cigarette smoking (increases the risk factor by 2 to 6)
• Hyperlipidemia-cholesterol levels greater than 200 (low-density lipoprotein greater than 120; high-density lipoprotein less than 35; triglycerides greater than 165)
• Obesity
• Sedentary lifestyle
• Stress
• Aggressive, competitive, hostile, chronically impatient

Other factors associated with increased risk include the following:
• Use of oral contraceptives
• Thyrotoxicosis
• Increase in levels of serum fibrinogen and uric acid
• Elevated hematocrit
• High heart rate when resting
• Reduced vital capacity

NURSE ALERT:
Patients may not recognize the signs of CAD. Fatigue, dyspnea, or indigestion associated with physical exertion may all be "angina equivalents."

CAD may be indicated if the patient has a history of the following:
- Angina (see Chapter 8, "Angina Pectoris")
- Myocardial infarction (see Chapter 9, "Myocardial Infarction")
- Congestive heart failure (see Chapter 12,"Congestive Heart Failure and Pulmonary Edema")
- Sudden cardiac death (see Chapter 33, "Cardiac Tamponade")
- Arrhythmias (see Chapter 32, "Cardiac Arrhythmias and Conduction Disturbances")
- Cardiomegaly
- Mitral insufficiency (see Chapter 14, "Mitral Insufficiency")
- Ventricular aneurysm (see Chapter 17, "Aneurysms: Abdominal, Thoracic, and Femoral")
- Cardiogenic shock (see Chapter 31, "Cardiogenic and Noncardiogenic Shock")

▲ Physical Findings:

Angina is the most frequent symptom of CAD. Episodes of angina generally follow physical activity, but excitement, overeating, or cold may also precipitate an attack. Angina may waken some patients from a sound sleep.

NURSE ALERT:
Remember, CAD is often symptomless. In women, angina symptoms may be atypical.

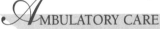

AMBULATORY CARE

When you assess an ambulatory patient for CAD, ask these questions:
- Do you tire more easily after physical activity?
- Do you ever feel short of breath when you exert yourself?
- Do you ever have pressure or pain in your chest, neck, jaw, arms, or back that is associated with activity?
- Have you ever undergone cardiac catheterization?
- Are you currently taking any heart medication?
- Have you ever been hospitalized because of your heart?

• Is your diet rich in
  - eggs (more than three egg yolks a week)?
  - red meat?
  - processed meat, including bacon?
  - whole milk products, including cheese, ice cream, and cream?
  - fried foods?
  - products processed in coconut or palm oil?
  - butter or lard?
  - hydrogenated fats?

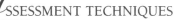

ASSESSMENT TECHNIQUES

Inspection, palpation, and auscultation can all reveal evidence of CAD.

You may discover the following symptoms upon inspection:
• Xanthelasma and xanthoma associated with elevated cholesterol levels; seen on eyelids as yellowish nodules
• Ophthalmoscopic examination shows an increase in light reflexes and arteriovenous nicking (seen in hypertensive patients)

You may discover the following symptoms upon palpation:
• Diminished peripheral pulses
• Edema in extremities with congestive heart failure

You may discover the following symptoms upon auscultation:
• Bruits
• S_3 or S_4
• Systolic murmur (mitral insufficiency)

Other indicators include the following:
• Chronic angina (particularly during exercise) that is relieved when the patient ceases physical activity or takes nitroglycerin indicates the onset of chronic CAD.
• Frequent angina that isn't relieved by rest or nitroglycerin or angina that occurs during sleep indicates the onset of acute CAD.

DIAGNOSTIC TESTS

TEST	FINDINGS
12-Lead (ECG)	• Ischemia • T-wave inversion • ST-segment depression • Arrhythmias 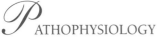 **NURSE ALERT:** Results may be normal during pain-free periods.
Treadmill or bicycle exercise tests or Persantine study	• Chest pain • ECG shows signs of myocardial ischemia
Myocardial perfusion imaging with treadmill	• Exercised-induced myocardial ischemia
Chest X-ray	• Cardiomegaly
Echocardiography	• Left ventricular akinesia or dyskinesia

𝒫ATHOPHYSIOLOGY

CAD starves the myocardial tissue of oxygen and nutrients as coronary blood flow diminishes. This occurs because fatty fibrous and/or calcium plaques narrow the coronary arteries. Ultimately, this can lead to myocardial infarction. Alternatively, the arteries may go into spasm, platelets aggregate, and a thrombus forms.

NURSE ALERT:
The patient is usually asymptomatic until 75% of an artery is blocked.

THE ATHEROSCLEROTIC PROCESS

Endothelial cells are mechanically
or chemically injured.

↓

Cell structures alter and become permeable to lipoproteins.
This is the first step in the development of CAD.

↓

The site of the injury attracts platelet aggregation and
adherence. It also attracts microphages.

↓

A fatty streak develops.
This is the second step in the development of CAD.

↓

Long-term injury causes a fibrofatty plaque.
This is the third step in the development of CAD.

↓

Deposits begin to invade the lumen.

↓

The vessel continues to narrow.

↓

Plaque can rupture, forming a thrombus and
further obstructing the artery.

↓

Coronary insufficiency results in myocardial ischemia.

*C*hapter 8. Angina Pectoris

▽ ▽ ▽ ▽ ▽ ▽ ▽

*I*NTRODUCTION

SEE TEXT PAGES

Angina pectoris is chest pain caused by myocardial ischemia. This occurs when blood flow into the heart does not meet metabolic demands or when the oxygen content of blood drops too low. Angina can be triggered by any level of physical activity, anxiety and stress, overeating, lying down to sleep, or cold temperatures.

*S*UPPORTING ASSESSMENT DATA

If your assessment findings are similar to those listed here, they may suggest angina pectoris.

▲ Health History:

In addition to all the health risk factors listed in Chapter 7, "Coronary Artery Disease," assess the patient for drug use, particularly amphetamines or cocaine, which cause excessive sympathetic stimulation and myocardial work.

Remember: Angina sufferers may describe sensations other than pain—that is, burning, aching, pressure, smothering, and symptoms associated with indigestion.

When you assess a patient for angina, ask these questions:
• What do you do that precipitates the pain?
• How would you describe the pain?
• Where does the pain/discomfort start and does it radiate?
• On a scale of 1 to 10, how would you rate your pain?
• Does anything help the pain/discomfort?
• How long does the pain/discomfort last and how often is it experienced?
• Do you carry nitroglycerin? If yes:
  – When did you last take it?
  – How many tablets relieve your symptoms?
  – How often do you use nitroglycerin in a given week?
• Do you take any other heart medications, such as beta blockers, calcium channel blockers, or nitrates?

▲ Physical Findings:

Angina pectoris may be indicated if the patient suffers from any of the symptoms listed in Chapter 7, "Coronary

Artery Disease." In addition, look for the following:
• Coronary artery spasm
• Aortic valve disease
• Anemia
• Aortitis

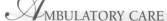

AMBULATORY CARE

Ask the ambulatory patient the following questions:
• Do you wear medical alert identification?
• Have you ever had cardiac catheterization? If yes, what were the results?
• Does your angina stop you from doing things? If yes, describe.

ASSESSMENT TECHNIQUES

You may discover the following symptoms upon inspection:
• Anxiety
• Fist clenched over sternum—pain is retrosternal or to the left of sternum

NURSE ALERT:
Pain can also occur on the right side.

• Nausea or vomiting
• Sweating
• Pallor
• Diaphoresis
• Dilation of pupils
• Distended neck veins
• Abnormal respiration

You may discover the following symptoms upon auscultation:
• Ventricular gallop (S_3)
• Atrial gallop (S_4)

Other indicators include the following:
• Complaint of toothache or jaw pain
• Pain in the left shoulder and upper arm that travels down the inside of the arm to the elbow, wrist, and fourth and fifth fingers
• Relief from nitroglycerin or rest
• Tachycardia
• Dyspnea
• Changes in blood pressure and pulse rate
• Dizziness or faintness
• Palpitations

DIAGNOSTIC TESTS

TEST	FINDINGS
Stress ECG	May be normal, or ST changes may be present
12-Lead ECG	May be normal; alternatively, may indicate myocardial ischemia by ST depression in affected areas
Cardiac isoenzyme levels	Normal
Coronary arteriography	Lesions, valvular disease
Echocardiography	May be normal; alternatively, may show hypertrophy, abnormal valve function, or abnormal wall motion

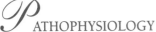ATHOPHYSIOLOGY

Angina pectoris occurs when a coronary artery narrows, reducing blood flow to the heart. Coronary artery disease (CAD) is the usual cause of angina pectoris. Occasionally, arterial spasm, not CAD, causes artery narrowing and angina. Angina pectoris resembles a heart attack; however, the pain is not as severe, it's of shorter duration, it diminishes with rest (reduced need for increased blood flow), and it doesn't cause permanent damage.

PATTERNS OF ANGINA

TYPE	PATTERN
Stable (classic)	Same amount of exertion or emotional stress triggers pain; predictable; no change over a period of months
Unstable (crescendo)	Differing degrees of exertion or emotional stress trigger pain; unpredictable; patient's normal anginal symptoms have increased in frequency and duration

PATTERNS OF ANGINA *(CONTINUED)*

TYPE	PATTERN
Variant (Prinzmetal's)	Similar to classic; lasts longer (up to 30 minutes), occurs with rest, appears in the early part of the day; may be caused by coronary artery spasm; appears in patients in their 30s and 40s and in heavy smokers
Nocturnal	Only occurs at night
Decubitus	Occurs when patient lies down; eases when patient sits or stands
Intractable	Chronic; incapacitates patient; does not respond to treatment
Postinfarction	Follows myocardial infarction; secondary to residual ischemia
Syndrome X	• Hard to diagnose; vessels in microvascular system fail to dilate correctly; primarily a disease of women (72%) from their 20s to age 65 • Pain is sharp, lasts 30 minutes or longer; the first episode is sudden; in later episodes, pain comes and goes

THE PATHOPHYSIOLOGY OF ANGINA

> Coronary arteries cannot supply enough blood to the heart in response to the demand due to CAD or spasm.

↓

> Within 10 seconds, myocardial cells experience ischemia.

↓

> Ischemic cells cannot obtain enough oxygen or glucose.

↓

> Ischemic myocardial cells may have reduced electrical and muscular function.

↓

> The cells convert to anaerobic metabolism.

↓

> The cells produce lactic acid as waste.

↓

> Pain develops from lactic acid accumulation.

↓

> Patient feels anginal symptoms until reducing demand decreases oxygen requirements of the myocardial cells.

Chapter 9. Myocardial Infarction

▽   ▽   ▽   ▽   ▽   ▽   ▽

INTRODUCTION

SEE TEXT PAGES

Myocardial infarction (MI) is a heart attack or coronary. It's extremely serious and is caused by the blockage of a coronary artery that robs the heart of oxygen and blood. Diagnosis and treatment within the first 48 hours are critical. Heart attacks are the leading cause of death, causing at least a half million fatalities a year in North America and Western Europe. More than half of those fatalities take place within 1 hour after the patient first experiences symptoms—usually before he or she gets to the emergency department. Even among those patients who survive, 10% die within a year.

SUPPORTING ASSESSMENT DATA

▼
▼
▼
▼
▼
▼
▼
▼
▼

If your assessment findings are similar to those listed here, they may suggest MI.

▲ Health History:

In addition to the health risk factors listed in Chapter 7, "Coronary Artery Disease," assess the patient for drug use, particularly amphetamines or cocaine, which cause sympathetic stimulation.

When you assess a patient for MI, ask these questions:
- Do you have a history of
  - Coronary artery spasm?
  - Coronary artery embolism?
  - Ventricular septal defect?
  - Systemic or pulmonary thromboembolism?
- What activities trigger the pain?
- Is the pain tight, constrictive, or choking?
- Where does the pain start? Does it radiate?
- Is it mild, moderate, or severe?
- Does anything help relieve the pain?
- How long does it last? How often do you have it?
- Have you ever had a previous heart attack? If yes,
  - Do you know where your heart was damaged?
  - Were you ever told you had a "silent" heart attack?
  - Have you ever taken "clot buster" medication?
  - Are you currently taking any heart medication?

▲ Physical Findings:

MI may be indicated if the patient suffers from any of the symptoms listed in Chapter 7, "Coronary Artery Disease." In addition, look for the following:

- Coronary artery spasm
- Coronary artery embolism
- Ventricular septal defect
- Systemic or pulmonary thromboembolism

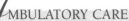

ⒶMBULATORY CARE

Ask the ambulatory patient these additional questions:
- Have you ever attended a cardiac rehabilitation program?
- Do you wear medical alert identification?
- Do you know how much heart damage you have?

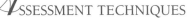

ⒶSSESSMENT TECHNIQUES

Inspection, palpation, and auscultation can all reveal MI. You may discover the following symptoms upon inspection:

- Anxiety, weakness, fear
- Complaints of chest pain or pressure that lasts longer than 30 minutes and is unrelieved by rest or nitroglycerin
- Nausea and/or vomiting
- Pain that travels to the neck, jaw, shoulder, back, or, most often, left arm
- Cyanosis
- Dyspnea, orthopnea

You may discover the following symptoms upon palpation:
- Cold, clammy, diaphoretic skin
- Thrills, heaves, abnormal point of maximum impulse
- Irregular, thready, or abnormally slow or fast pulse

You may discover the following symptoms upon auscultation:
- Bruits
- Ventricular gallop (S_3)
- Atrial gallop (S_4)
- Pericardial friction rub
- Crackles
- Systolic murmur (mitral insufficiency)

Other indicators include the following:
- Fear of death
- Hypotension
- Lethargy
- Palpitations
- Shock
- Fever

NURSE ALERT:
Some patients, especially diabetics or elderly patients, may have no pain or the pain is so mild it's mistaken for indigestion. Among middle-aged men, 10% have no pain. Consider any patient with three or more risk factors at risk for a "silent" heart attack.

DIAGNOSTIC TESTS

The following table lists general diagnostic findings with MI. Remember: You must see changes in at least two leads of the 12-lead ECG. Lateral precordial leads usually show Q-wave changes. ECG may appear normal up to a few hours after MI.

TEST	FINDINGS
ECG	• Leads directed toward the infarction show pathologic Q waves at least 0.04 seconds (1 mm) wide and a quarter of the QRS complex height. • Leads over or directed toward the infarction show elevated ST changes. • Leads 180 degrees from infarction show ST-segment depression (reciprocal changes). • During initial infarction, leads over the infarcted area may show peaked, upright T waves. • Where ST-segment elevation is present, T wave is usually inverted. • ST segment becomes isoelectric after a few hours or even days. T wave often stays inverted.
Complete blood count	Increased leukocytes
Erythrocyte sedimentation rate	Elevated

DIAGNOSTIC TESTS (CONTINUED)

TEST	FINDINGS
Creatine kinase (CK)	• Shows increase at 4 to 6 hours; peaks within 12 to 24 hours; elevation lasts as long as 3 days • May be present with other conditions
Lactate dehydrogenase (LDH)	• Shows increase at 8 to 12 hours; peaks within 2 to 4 days; elevation lasts as long as 14 days • May be present with other conditions
CK-MB isoenzymes	Indicative of MI; if 4% greater than total CK, diagnose MI
LDH isoenzymes	LDH_1 elevated and LDH_1-LDH_2 ratio greater than 1
Coronary angiography	• Stenosis • Occlusion
Arterial blood gas analysis	• Hypoxemia (drop in Pao_2) • Hyperventilation (drop in $Paco_2$)
Chest X-ray	• Cardiomegaly • Left ventricular failure—pulmonary congestion

PINPOINTING MI TRIGGER LOCATIONS

LOCATION	TEST	FINDINGS
Ischemia	• Serial 12-lead ECG	• Depression of ST segment—possibly in all leads • Inverted T wave—possibly in all leads
Anterior infarction	• Serial 12-lead ECG	• Changes in leads V_{1-4} • Leads II, III, and aVF show reciprocal changes
Anterolateral infarction	• Serial 12-lead ECG	• Leads I, aVL, and V_{4-6} show Q wave and inverted T wave • Leads V_{1-6} show changes
Anteroseptal infarction	• Serial 12-lead ECG	• Leads V_{1-4} show changes
Subendocardial injury (damage to innermost layer of myocardial tissue)	• Serial 12-lead ECG	• No abnormal Q waves (myocardium still partially electroactive) • Leads directed toward epicardial surface over infarction area show ST-segment depression and inverted T waves • Greater than 1-mm elevation of ST segment and T wave that becomes normal with cessation of pain
	• Hemodynamic monitoring in CCU	• Abnormal cardiac output and pulmonary artery pressure that suggests serious injury

PINPOINTING MI TRIGGER LOCATIONS (CONTINUED)

LOCATION	TEST	FINDINGS
Subepicardial injury	• Serial 12-lead ECG	• Elevation of ST segment and T wave indicative of Prinzmetal's angina; often appears before MI
	• Hemodynamic monitoring in CCU	• Abnormal cardiac output and pulmonary artery pressure that suggests serious injury
Right ventrical infarction	• Serial 12-lead ECG	• Changes in right precordial chest leads • Leads V_{4-6} show ST elevation
Diaphragmatic (inferior) infarction	• Serial 12-lead ECG	• Leads II, III, aVF, and, at times, lateral precordial show ST-T changes • Leads I, aVL, and precordial leads of anterior chest show reciprocal changes
Posterior wall infarction	• Serial 12-lead ECG • No reflection of posterior surface of heart on any lead	• Anterior chest leads V_{1-3} show reciprocal changes • V_1 and V_2 show unusually tall R waves • Leads V_{1-3} show ST-segment depression and tall T waves
Defect in right and left ventricular wall motion	• Radiopharmaceutical imaging scans • Multiple-gated acquisition scan • Echocardiogram	• Location of left ventricular damage • Defect in motion; also shows aneurysms • Right ventricular infarcts, cavity size, decrease in performance, and abnormal wall motion as a result of MI damage

PATHOPHYSIOLOGY

Coronary artery blockage resulting from atherosclerosis or coronary artery spasm or hemorrhage into a plaque can cause MI. Once blood flow ceases, myocardial tissue dies. You can detect signs of ischemia within 8 to 10 seconds of the cessation of blood flow. Cellular death occurs after 20 minutes of sustained ischemia. The myocardial cells revert to anaerobic metabolism and begin to produce lactic acid. This causes the myocardial cells to lose function; thus, you will see symptoms of abnormal conduction, arrhythmias, and a loss of contractility.

The most common sites of infarction are as follows:
- Anterior wall of left ventricle in vicinity of apex
- Posterior wall of left ventricle in vicinity of base
- Inferior surface of the heart muscle

Specific terminology for describing the areas of infarction includes the following (refer to illustration below):
- Zone of infarction—actual infarcted site
- Zone of hypoxic injury—area of injury around the infarcted site can heal, but necrosis is likely if you cannot restore blood flow
- Zone of ischemia—possible to prevent damage to this area

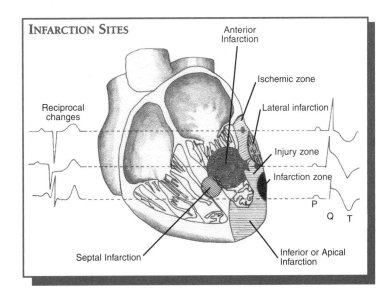

INFARCTION SITES

Anterior Infarction

Ischemic zone

Reciprocal changes

Lateral infarction

Injury zone

Infarction zone

P

Q   T

Septal Infarction

Inferior or Apical Infarction

INFARCTION SITES AND BLOCKED VESSELS

OCCLUDED VESSEL	INFARCTION SITE
Left main artery	• Large anterior wall • Large anterior septal wall • Large anterior lateral wall Associated with • Sudden cardiac death • Congestive heart failure
Left circumflex artery	• Lateral wall • Inferolateral wall • Posterior wall
Left anterior coronary artery	• Anterior wall • Septal wall • Apical wall Associated with • Right bundle branch block and left anterior hemiblock • Mobitz type II heart block • Complete heart block • Congestive heart failure • Hypotension
Right coronary artery	• Inferior wall • Right ventricle Associated with • First-degree block • Mobitz type I heart block • Second-degree heart block • Bradycardia • Hypotension

Chapter 10. Cardiomyopathy

▽ ▽ ▽ ▽ ▽ ▽ ▽

INTRODUCTION

SEE TEXT PAGES

Cardiomyopathy is a disorder of the heart muscle that may be chronic or subacute. Its source is often difficult to identify.

SUPPORTING ASSESSMENT DATA

If your assessment findings are similar to those listed here, they may suggest cardiomyopathy.

▲ **Health History:**

In addition to the health risk factors listed in Chapter 7, "Coronary Artery Disease," consider possible cardiomyopathy in patients who are:
• Pregnant or post partum
• Alcoholic
• Immobile and confined to a bed
• In congestive heart failure
• In atrial fibrillation

Also find out if patients have or have had the following:
• A family history of cardiomyopathy
• An endocrine disorder
• A dilated myocardium
• An infection

▲ **Physical Findings:**

Cardiomyopathy may be indicated if the patient has any of the following symptoms:
• Fatigue and weakness
• Chest pain
• Exercise intolerance
• Ascites
• Dyspnea on exertion
• Angina-like pain
• Fainting

NURSE ALERT:
Death can occur without warning, especially if the patient is a child or young adult.

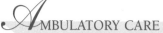

AMBULATORY CARE

When you assess an ambulatory patient, ask these questions:
• Do you wear medical alert identification?
• Are you involved in any experimental drug protocols?
• Has heart transplantation ever been discussed with you?
• Have ventricular assist devices or dynamic cardiomy-oplasty been discussed with you?
• Do you take any heart medications?
• Do you take Coumadin?

ASSESSMENT TECHNIQUES

You may discover the following symptoms upon inspection:
• Anxiety
• Irritability
• CNS symptoms, including confusion and somnolence
• Restlessness
• Irritability
• Pallor
• Diaphoresis
• Dilation of pupils
• Distended neck veins
• Dyspnea
• Abnormal respiration

Other indicators include the following:
• Hypercapnia
• Hypoxia
• Inability to remove secretions
• Anorexia
• Tachycardia
• Tachypnea
• Hemoptysis
• Orthopnea
• Dizziness or faintness
• Decreased blood pressure
• Increased heart rate and respiratory rate
• Elevated pulmonary artery pressure

CLASSES OF CARDIOMYOPATHY

There are three classes of cardiomyopathy: dilated or congestive (cardiac enlargement), hypertrophic (thickening of the interventricular septum), and restrictive (rigid ventricular walls). The following table describes the results of palpation, percussion, and auscultation for each class.

CLASS	PALPATION	PERCUSSION	AUSCULTATION
Dilated	• Enlarged liver • Narrow pulse pressure • Pulsus alternans dull • Cool skin • Jugular vein distention • Laterally displaced point of maximum impulse • Left ventricular heave • Peripheral edema	• Cardiac enlargement • Bases of lungs dull	• Irregular heartbeat • S_3 and S_4 heart sound • Murmurs • Mitral and tricuspid insufficiency • Crackles
Hypertrophic	• Displaced apical impulse • Systolic thrill		• S_4 heart sound • Possibly S_3 heart sound • Split S_2 heart sound • Systolic ejection murmur
Restrictive	• Ascites • Edema • Positive hepatojugular reflex (HJR) • Right upper quadrant pain	• Cardiac enlargement • Pulmonary congestion	• S_3 and S_4 heart sounds • Mitral and tricuspid insufficiency

DIAGNOSTIC TESTS

TEST	FINDINGS
Chest X-ray	• Increased heart size • Pulmonary hypertension
12-Lead ECG	• Left ventricular hypertrophy • Conduction defects • Left atrial and ventricular enlargement • Nonspecific ST-segment changes • T-wave abnormalities • Leads II, III, aVF, and V_{4-6} show Q waves similar to those seen with an infarction • Left anterior hemiblock • Left axis deviation • Arrhythmias
Radiopharmaceutical imaging scans	• Myocardial perfusion defects
Cardiac catheterization	• Elevated left ventricular end-diastolic, pulmonary capillary wedge pressure, and pulmonary artery pressure with decreasing cardiac output • Elevated right ventricular end-diastolic, right atrial, and central venous pressures • Mitral insufficiency • Rarely, left atrium is shaped like a slipper and left ventricle like a spade
Echocardiography	• Thickening of ventricular walls • Septal thickening • Elevated end-systolic and end-diastolic volumes • Anterior mitral leaflet moves abnormally during systole • Chamber restriction of left ventricle • Poor contractility

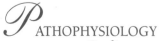

PATHOPHYSIOLOGY

Cardiomyopathy is a disease of the heart muscle. It can involve the endocardial and pericardial layers. Its cause is usually unknown, but at least 50% of cases are inherited.

THE PROGRESSION OF CARDIOMYOPATHY

TYPE	CHARACTERIZATION
Dilated or congestive (most common)	• Degeneration of myocardial fibers • Increase in fibrotic tissue • Dilation of all four chambers, particularly ventricles • First symptom is contractile dysfunction • Mitral insufficiency • Progressive deterioration of heart muscle due to toxic, metabolic, or infectious causes • Congestive heart failure • Death
Hypertrophic	• Hypertrophied left ventricle with no increase in cavity size • May have restricted filling and outflow obstruction, referred to as hypertrophic obstructive cardiomyopathy; causes increased left atrial and ventricular pressures • Rigidity develops in ventricles • Left ventricle loses compliance (cardiac output may be high, low, or normal) • Decompensation occurs, sometimes quickly or sometimes over a long period of time. Cardiac death may occur with no previous symptoms.
Restrictive (least common)	• Myocardium, endocardium, and subendocardium infiltrated • Restrictive ventricular filling, loss of distention, and contraction during systole and diastole • Left ventricular end-diastolic pressure increases • Cardiac output drops—congestive heart failure and death

Chapter 11. Hypertension

▽   ▽   ▽   ▽   ▽   ▽   ▽

INTRODUCTION

SEE TEXT PAGES

Hypertension is characterized by an intermittent or a sustained diastolic pressure above 90 mm Hg and systolic pressure above 140 mm Hg. It's a serious condition that is potentially life-threatening.

SUPPORTING ASSESSMENT DATA

If your assessment findings are similar to those listed here, they may suggest hypertension.

▲ Health History:

In addition to the health risk factors listed in Chapter 7, "Coronary Artery Disease," consider at risk patients to whom the following conditions apply:

- Men
- Black (two times more at risk than whites, four times more likely to die)
- Toxemia of pregnancy
- Suffering from pituitary tumors
- Suffering from coarctation of the aorta
- Using catecholamine precursors and monoamine oxidase inhibitors
- Suffering from adrenocortical hyperfunction
- Suffering from Cushing's syndrome
- Alcoholic
- Ingesting high levels of sodium
- Suffering from atherosclerosis
- Suffering from renal disease
- Suffering from polycythemia
- From a family with a history of hypertension
- Over age 40
- In atrial fibrillation
- Suffering from a dilated myocardium
- Suffering from an infection

If the patient is known to have hypertension, ask these questions:

- When were you told you had high blood pressure?
- Are you currently taking any blood pressure medication?
- Do you take any diuretics?
- Have you recently stopped or run out of any medications?
- Do you frequently eat canned, Chinese, or other salty food?
- Do you smoke? If so, how much?
- How much exercise do you do regularly?
- How much caffeine do you consume in a day?
- Do you have kidney disease or diabetes?
- Have you ever had a stroke or ministroke?

▲ Physical Findings:

Hypertension often causes no symptoms. Usually, it's diagnosed during a physical examination or other evaluation. Symptoms are the result of the impact of hypertension on organ systems. When symptoms are present, patients complain of the following:
- Chest pain
- Dizziness and fainting
- Visual abnormalities
- Vomiting
- Transient paralysis
- Nosebleeds
- Fatigue
- Seizures
- Stupor
- Tinnitus
- Palpitations
- Impotence
- Occipital headaches
- Dyspnea (left ventricular hypertrophy)
- Nocturia (renal insufficiency)
- Cerebellar changes, including stroke or hemorrhage (cerebrovascular disease)

NURSE ALERT:
If chest pain or dyspnea is present, suspect coronary artery disease.

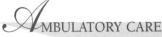

AMBULATORY CARE

Ask ambulatory patients:
- Do you wear medical alert identification?

ASSESSMENT TECHNIQUES

You may discover the following symptoms upon inspection:
- Anxiety
- Flushing
- Peripheral edema (heart failure)
- Ophthalmoscopic examination may reveal hemorrhages, exudate, papilledema (hypertensive retinopathy), increased light reflex, and other changes in optic fundi (retinopathy)
- Labored respiration

You may discover the following symptoms upon palpation:
- Decreased or absent carotid pulse
- Presence of pulsating mass (possible abdominal aneurysm)
- Enlarged kidneys

You may discover the following symptoms upon auscultation:
- Abdominal bruit
- Renal bruit
- Bruits over abdominal aorta
- Bruits over femoral aorta
- Systolic murmur

DIAGNOSTIC TESTS

TEST	FINDINGS
Chest X-ray	Useful in only 2% of cases (enlarged heart)
12-Lead ECG	• Left ventricular hypertrophy • Ischemia
Urinalysis	• Protein, red blood cells, or white blood cells (renal disease) • Glucose (diabetes)

DIAGNOSTIC TESTS (CONTINUED)

TEST	FINDINGS
Excretory urography	• Renal atrophy (chronic renal disease) • One enlarged kidney (unilateral renal disease)
Serum potassium	Lower than 3.5 mEq/liter (adrenal dysfunction)
Blood urea nitrogen	Normal or elevated to greater than 20 mg/dL with serum creatinine levels listed below (renal disease)
Serum creatinine	Normal or elevated to more than 1.5 mg/dL

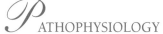

ATHOPHYSIOLOGY

Hypertension is a serious health problem. Its presence predisposes a patient to heart attack, renal failure, stroke, blindness, cerebral hemorrhage, and death. These signs manifest themselves after the patient has had hypertension for an extended period of time.

Hypertension can influence any organ system but most often affects the heart, brain, eyes, and kidneys. Over time, it can cause atherosclerosis (plaque formation) in the arteries of the heart, brain, and kidneys as well as aneurysm and hyaline and hyperplastic arteriosclerosis.

Blood pressure is the pressure of blood flow on artery walls. Mean arterial pressure is a function of cardiac output and systemic vascular resistance.

When the patient's diastolic pressure ranges from 90 to 104, the hypertension is mild. If it ranges from 105 to 114, hypertension is moderate. If it's over 115, consider the hypertension severe.

CLASSIFYING HYPERTENSION

Hypertension is classified as essential, secondary, or malignant. The following table describes the differences among these classifications.

CLASSIFICATION	CHARACTERIZATION
Essential	More than 90% of cases; no cause; no symptoms in early stages; treatment consists of controlling symptoms
Secondary	Caused by a disease, medication, or other etiology; treatment consists of treating the underlying cause
Malignant	End product of untreated essential or secondary hypertension; life-threatening; diastolic pressure rapidly rises above 120 mm Hg

THE PROGRESSION OF UNCONTROLLED HYPERTENSION

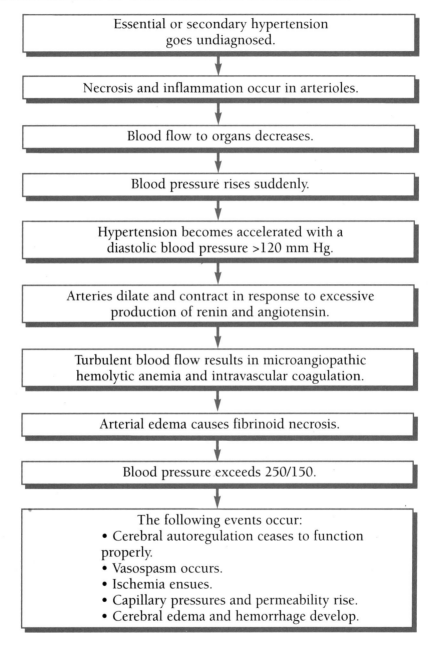

Essential or secondary hypertension
goes undiagnosed.

↓

Necrosis and inflammation occur in arterioles.

↓

Blood flow to organs decreases.

↓

Blood pressure rises suddenly.

↓

Hypertension becomes accelerated with a
diastolic blood pressure >120 mm Hg.

↓

Arteries dilate and contract in response to excessive
production of renin and angiotensin.

↓

Turbulent blood flow results in microangiopathic
hemolytic anemia and intravascular coagulation.

↓

Arterial edema causes fibrinoid necrosis.

↓

Blood pressure exceeds 250/150.

↓

The following events occur:
• Cerebral autoregulation ceases to function
properly.
• Vasospasm occurs.
• Ischemia ensues.
• Capillary pressures and permeability rise.
• Cerebral edema and hemorrhage develop.

Chapter 12. Congestive Heart Failure and Pulmonary Edema

▽   ▽   ▽   ▽   ▽   ▽   ▽

INTRODUCTION

SEE TEXT PAGES

Congestive heart failure (CHF) occurs when the heart can no longer provide the body with adequate oxygen or nutrients. Pulmonary edema is a serious condition in which the alveoli develop severe edema.

SUPPORTING ASSESSMENT DATA

If your assessment findings are similar to those listed here, they may suggest CHF or pulmonary edema.

▲ **Health History:**

In addition to the health risk factors listed in Chapter 7, "Coronary Artery Disease," consider at risk patients who have a history of the following:

- Cardiomyopathy
- Congenital heart defects
- Systemic hypertension
- Pulmonary hypertension
- Myocardial infarction (MI)
- Valvular stenosis or insufficiency
- Cardiac tamponade
- Constrictive pericarditis
- Hypervolemia
- Coronary artery disease
- Generalized tonic-clonic seizures (pulmonary edema)
- Head trauma (pulmonary edema)

In addition, consider at risk patients who have the following:

- Arrhythmias
- Extreme physical and emotional stress
- Infection
- Anemia
- Thyroid disease
- Pulmonary disease
- Any other chronic illness, such as kidney disease

Ask these questions as part of the health history for a patient diagnosed with heart failure:
- Do you take any heart medication?
- Have you recently stopped taking or run out of any medications?
- Have you recently changed your diet? Do you eat out often?
- Are you enrolled in any experimental drug protocols?
- Has heart transplantation ever been discussed with you?
- Have ventricular assist devices or dynamic cardiomyoplasty been discussed with you?
- Do you use oxygen at home?
- Do you take any diuretics?
- Are you on a program of sodium and fluid restriction?
- Are you on a special diet?
- Do you have to sit up to sleep?
- Do you practice emotional and physical stress reduction?
- Do you take ACE (angiotensin-converting enzyme) inhibitors like captopril?
- Do you have kidney disease or diabetes?

▲ Physical Findings:

Both CHF and pulmonary edema present with symptoms. Patients complain of the following symptoms:
- Chest pain or discomfort
- Shortness of breath
- Orthopnea
- Diaphoresis
- Oliguria
- Confusion
- Nocturia
- Nocturnal dyspnea
- Anorexia
- Weight gain
- Edema
- Fatigue and weakness

AMBULATORY CARE

When you assess the ambulatory patient, ask these questions:
- Do you wear medical alert identification?
- How often have you been hospitalized for heart failure?
- Do you know your ejection fraction (or heart's pumping ability percentage)?
- Does your heart failure limit your lifestyle? If yes, how?

COMMON CHF ASSESSMENT FINDINGS

TECHNIQUE	LEFT VENTRICULAR FAILURE	RIGHT VENTRICULAR FAILURE
Inspection	• Anxiety • Confusion • Productive cough (frothy or bloody) • Abnormal respiration • Weakness and fatigue • Anorexia • Pale, dusky skin • Cyanosis • Pulsus alternans • Weight gain	• Kussmaul's sign • Distended jugular vein when sitting • Weight gain • Nausea and gastric distress • Peripheral edema • Weakness and fatigue • Anorexia • Pale, dusky skin • Cyanosis • Pulsus alternans
Palpation	• Point of maximal impulse enlarged • Diaphoresis • Liver enlargement • Ascites • Edema (pitting)	• Abdominal edema (ascites) • Enlarged spleen • Damp skin • Liver enlargement • Edema (pitting)
Auscultation	• Mitral insufficiency murmur • Ventricular gallop (S_3) • Atrial gallop (S_4) • Crackles	• Tricuspid insufficiency murmur • Kussmaul's sign • Bounding pulse • Ventricular gallop (S_3) • Atrial gallop (S_4) • Crackles
Other findings	• Premature atrial contractions • Orthopnea • Nocturnal dyspnea • Nocturia • Tachycardia • Tachypnea • Hypotension	• Abdominal pain • Tachycardia • Tachypnea • Hypotension

DIAGNOSTIC TESTS

TEST	FINDINGS
Chest X-ray	• Enlarged heart • Engorged pulmonary vasculature
12-Lead ECG	• Old anterior or anterior septal MI damage; current ischemic changes
Arterial blood gas analysis	• Hypoxia
Serum enzymes	• Elevated aspartate transaminase (formerly serum glutamic-oxaloacetic transaminase) due to enlarged liver
Serum electrolytes	• Hyponatremia (dilutional) • Hyperkalemia (decreased glomerular filtration) • Hypokalemia (diuretics)
Serum bilirubin	• Hyperbilirubinemia (enlarged liver)
Complete blood count	• Decreased hemoglobin and hematocrit (anemia)

CAUSES OF RIGHT AND LEFT VENTRICULAR FAILURE AND PULMONARY EDEMA

LEFT VENTRICULAR FAILURE	RIGHT VENTRICULAR FAILURE	PULMONARY EDEMA
• Acute MI of left ventricle • Cardiomyopathy • Increased circulating volume • Aortic stenosis • Cardiac tamponade • Constrictive pericarditis • Atherosclerosis • Tachycardia • Bradycardia • Ventricular septal defect • Mitral stenosis	• Acute MI of right ventricle • Pulmonary embolism • Left ventricular failure • Fluid overload • Excess sodium intake • Atrial defect • Pulmonary outflow stenosis • Obstructive pulmonary disease • Atherosclerosis • Bradycardia • Ventricular septal defect • Mitral stenosis • Tachycardia	• Left ventricular failure • Hypertension • CNS disorders • Volume overload

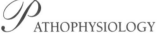ATHOPHYSIOLOGY

CHF is not a disease in itself but reflects myocardial tissue dysfunction, resulting in pump failure. Decreased contractility can be caused by direct damage from a recent MI, or from chronic conditions that have strained the heart muscle, such as valvular stenosis or insufficiency and hypertension.

Decreased cardiac output means that the metabolic needs or oxygen consumption of vital organs cannot be met. The symptoms you will assess are the result of poor ventricular performance.

Pulmonary edema occurs when the alveoli and extravascular spaces in the lung are flooded with fluid. Left ventricular failure is the most common cause of pulmonary edema, but other conditions that create an imbalance between hydrostatic pressure and colloid osmotic pressure in the pulmonary capillaries can also cause pulmonary edema.

THE PATHOPHYSIOLOGY OF CHF

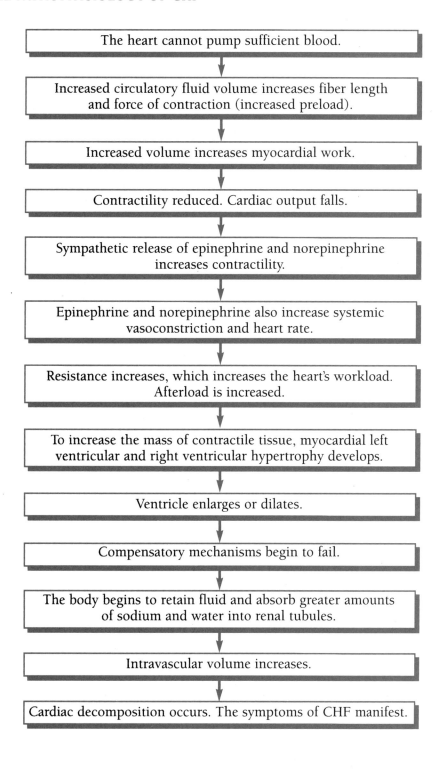

The heart cannot pump sufficient blood.

↓

Increased circulatory fluid volume increases fiber length and force of contraction (increased preload).

↓

Increased volume increases myocardial work.

↓

Contractility reduced. Cardiac output falls.

↓

Sympathetic release of epinephrine and norepinephrine increases contractility.

↓

Epinephrine and norepinephrine also increase systemic vasoconstriction and heart rate.

↓

Resistance increases, which increases the heart's workload. Afterload is increased.

↓

To increase the mass of contractile tissue, myocardial left ventricular and right ventricular hypertrophy develops.

↓

Ventricle enlarges or dilates.

↓

Compensatory mechanisms begin to fail.

↓

The body begins to retain fluid and absorb greater amounts of sodium and water into renal tubules.

↓

Intravascular volume increases.

↓

Cardiac decomposition occurs. The symptoms of CHF manifest.

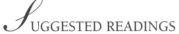

SUGGESTED READINGS

Anardi, D. M. "Assessment of Right Heart Function." *Journal of Cardiovascular Nursing* 6 (1991): 12–33.

Berczeller, P. H. "Congestive Heart Failure and Bradycardia." *Hospital Practice* 29 (January 15, 1994): 111–114.

Goldman, H. "Myocardial Infarction, Diagnosis and Treatment." *Nursing Times* 90 (1994): 33–37.

Hertzeanu, H. L. "Ventricular Arrhythmias in Rehabilitated and Nonrehabilitated Post-Myocardial Infarction Patients with LV Dysfunction." *American Journal of Cardiology* 71 (January 1, 1993): 24–27.

Lavie, C. J. "Factors Predicting Improvements in Lipid Values Following Cardiac Rehabilitation and Exercise Training." *Archives of Internal Medicine* 153 (1993): 982–988.

Swearingen, P. L. *Manual of Medical Surgical Nursing Care.* St. Louis: Mosby Year Book, Inc., 1994.

Van Buskirk, M. C., and A. H. Gradman. "Monitoring Blood Pressure in Ambulatory Patients." *AJN* 93 (1993): 44–47.

SECTION IV: VALVULAR HEART DISEASE

$\mathscr{C}$hapter 13. Mitral Stenosis

▽ ▽ ▽ ▽ ▽ ▽ ▽

$\mathscr{I}$NTRODUCTION

SEE TEXT PAGES

Mitral stenosis occurs when the mitral orifice develops an obstruction to blood flow. The left atrium (LA) and left ventricle (LV) fail to receive an adequate amount of blood during diastolic movement.

$\mathscr{S}$UPPORTING ASSESSMENT DATA

▼
▼
▼
▼
▼
▼
▼
▼
▼
▼

If your assessment findings are similar to those listed here, they may suggest mitral stenosis.

▲ Health History:

In addition to the health risk factors listed in Chapter 7, "Coronary Artery Disease," consider at risk patients with a history of the following:
• Rheumatic heart disease
• Congenital heart disease
• Gradual decline in physical activity
• Repeated respiratory infections

In addition, consider women in their early 30s at risk.

▲ Physical Findings:

Patients with moderate to severe mitral stenosis may complain of the following symptoms:
• Dyspnea on exertion
• Chest pain
• Progressive fatigue
• Cough
• Orthopnea
• Palpitations
• Symptoms of right ventricle (RV) failure (see Chapter 12, "Congestive Heart Failure and Pulmonary Edema")
• Dysphagia

NURSE ALERT:
If mitral stenosis is mild, the patient may be asymptomatic.

AMBULATORY CARE

When you assess the ambulatory patient with known mitral stenosis, ask these questions:
- Do you wear medical alert identification?
- Do you take Coumadin?
- Do you have a prescription for antibiotics?
- Have you ever had valve surgery?
- If yes, what type (commissurotomy, balloon valvuloplasty)? Did you have a valve replacement (pericardial tissue or artificial, such as a St. Jude valve)?
- Do you take heart medications?
- Do you have tumors in the left atrium?
- Do you have calcification of the mitral annulus?

ASSESSMENT TECHNIQUES

Use inspection, palpation, and auscultation to assess the patient.

The following findings are likely to be evident upon inspection:
- Ruddy cheeks
- Bloody, productive cough
- Peripheral edema
- Anorexia

The following findings are likely to be evident upon palpation:
- RV lift (pulmonary hypertension)
- Normal LV impulse
- Enlarged liver
- Decreased arterial pulse volume
- Thrill over apical area

The following findings are likely to be evident upon auscultation:
- Tricuspid insufficiency murmur (if RV failure present)
- Point of maximum impulse displacement (listen at mitral area, fifth intercostal space, midclavicular line)
- Diastolic murmur (extremely low)
- Pulmonary crackles
- S_1 accentuated with opening snap
- Pulmonary insufficiency murmur (if pulmonary hypertension present)

DIAGNOSTIC TESTS

TEST	FINDINGS
Chest X-ray	• LA and RV hypertrophy • Left border straightening • Pulmonary arteries enlarged • Interstitial edema • Dilated upper lobe pulmonary veins • Calcification of mitral valve
Cardiac catheterization	• Valve shows diastolic pressure gradient • LA and pulmonary artery pressures >15 mm Hg • Severe pulmonary hypertension • Calcification of mitral valve • Elevated RV pressure • Decreased cardiac output • Abnormal LV contraction
Echocardiography	• Thickening of anterior and posterior mitral valve leaflets • Abnormal leaflet movement • Enlargement of LA • Enlargement of RV
12-Lead ECG	• LA hypertrophy • Atrial fibrillation • RV hypertrophy • Right axis deviation

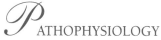

PATHOPHYSIOLOGY

Mitral stenosis is most often preceded by rheumatic fever. If the patient has no history of rheumatic fever, suspect a virus, a tumor, or congenital abnormalities.

NURSE ALERT:
Patients with mitral stenosis can be prone to endocarditis. Patients who must have surgery, including dental work, may require antibiotics.

THE PROGRESSION OF MITRAL STENOSIS

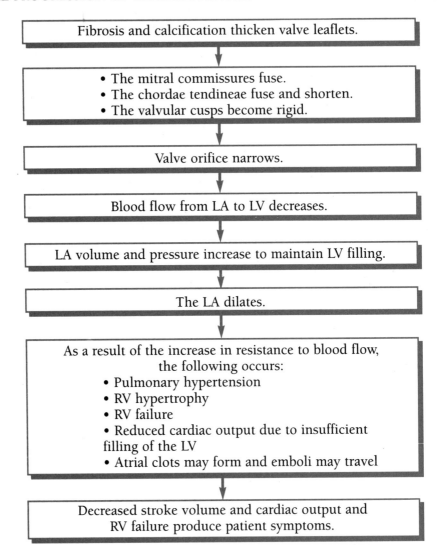

Fibrosis and calcification thicken valve leaflets.

- The mitral commissures fuse.
- The chordae tendineae fuse and shorten.
- The valvular cusps become rigid.

Valve orifice narrows.

Blood flow from LA to LV decreases.

LA volume and pressure increase to maintain LV filling.

The LA dilates.

As a result of the increase in resistance to blood flow, the following occurs:
- Pulmonary hypertension
- RV hypertrophy
- RV failure
- Reduced cardiac output due to insufficient filling of the LV
- Atrial clots may form and emboli may travel

Decreased stroke volume and cardiac output and RV failure produce patient symptoms.

Chapter 14. Mitral Insufficiency

▽   ▽   ▽   ▽   ▽   ▽   ▽

INTRODUCTION

SEE TEXT PAGES

Mitral insufficiency, or mitral regurgitation, is caused during systole by blood from the left ventricle (LV) flowing back into the left atrium (LA). This happens when the mitral valve is damaged.

SUPPORTING ASSESSMENT DATA

If your assessment findings are similar to those listed here, they may suggest mitral insufficiency.

▲ Health History:

In addition to the health risk factors listed in Chapter 7, "Coronary Artery Disease," consider at risk patients who have a history of the following:

- Trauma
- Rheumatic valvular disease
- Endocarditis
- Recent myocardial infarction or a family history of congenital defects of the mitral valve, chordae tendineae, or mitral ring
- Marfan's syndrome
- Streptococcal infection
- Ischemia
- Calcification (in older patients)
- Prolapsed mitral valve
- LV dilation
- Cardiomyopathy

▲ Physical Findings:

Patients with mitral insufficiency may complain of the following symptoms:

- Chest pain or discomfort
- Orthopnea
- Exertional dyspnea
- Anorexia
- Fatigue and weakness
- Palpitations

NURSE ALERT:
Patients may be asymptomatic.

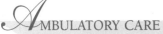

MBULATORY CARE

When you assess the ambulatory patient, ask these questions:
- Do you wear medical alert identification?
- Do you take any heart medication?
- Do you take Coumadin?
- Do you have a prescription for antibiotics?
- Have you ever had valve surgery? If yes, was it balloon valvuloplasty, commissurotomy, or a valve replacement (pericardial tissue or artificial, such as St. Jude)?

NURSE ALERT:
Patient may require antibiotics before any dental work.

SSESSMENT TECHNIQUES

Use inspection, palpation, percussion, and auscultation to assess the patient.

You may discover the following symptoms upon inspection:
- Anxiety
- Dyspnea
- Diaphoresis
- Cyanosis
- Jugular vein distention
- Peripheral edema (heart failure)
- Abnormal respiration

You may discover the following symptoms upon palpation:
- Chest—regular pulse with sharp upstroke
- Irregular pulse if patient has atrial fibrillation
- Systolic thrill
- Right ventricular (RV) tap at the apex (if pulmonary hypertension present)
- LA enlarged
- Enlarged liver (RV failure)

You may discover lateral cardiac border (dilated heart) on percussion.

You may discover the following symptoms upon auscultation:
- Soft S_1
- Systolic murmur
- Crackles in lungs (pulmonary congestion or edema)
- Holosystolic murmur—extremely indicative of mitral insufficiency; listen at the apex
- Split S_2
- Low S_3, sometimes followed by diastolic murmur; may hear S_4
- S_4 with recent onset of mitral insufficiency and normal sinus rhythm

DIAGNOSTIC TESTS

TEST	FINDINGS
Chest X-ray	• LA and LV enlargement • Pulmonary venous congestion • Mitral leaflet calcification
12-Lead ECG	• LA hypertrophy • LV hypertrophy • Sinus tachycardia • Atrial fibrillation
Echocardiography	• Abnormal motion of valve leaflets • LA enlargement • Mitral valve prolapse • Mitral annular calcification • Flail mitral leaflet • Vegetations • Regional wall motion abnormalities (papillary muscle dysfunction) • Hyperdynamic, enlarged LV
Cardiac catheterization	• Flow from LV to LA during systole (mitral insufficiency) • Elevated LV end-diastolic volume and pressure • Regurgitant fraction • Decreased cardiac output • Elevated LA pressure • Elevated pulmonary capillary wedge pressure (chronic mitral insufficiency)

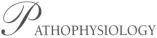ATHOPHYSIOLOGY

Mitral insufficiency tends to be progressive. It can be life-threatening. The following flowchart illustrates its pathophysiology.

A preexisting chronic or acute disorder damages
the mitral valve.

↓

Mitral valve becomes incompetent and
does not close properly during systole.

↓

LV regurgitates as much as 50% of stroke volume into LA.

↓

With acute onset:
- LA pressure increases.
- Pulmonary edema occurs.
- LV loses function and LV end-diastolic pressure rises.
- Pulmonary hypertension occurs.
- Pulmonary vascular bed compresses.
- Without treatment, the patient dies.

↓

With chronic onset:
- LA dilates.
- LA pressure slowly increases.
- LV compensates for chronic volume overload with dilation.
- Hypertrophy ensues.
- Pulmonary venous pressures elevate.
- Pulmonary hypertension occurs.
- Dilation causes arrhythmias (ventricular and atrial fibrillation).
- Without treatment, LV or RV failure occurs.
- Pulmonary edema occurs and cardiovascular collapse may occur.

Chapter 15. Aortic Stenosis

▽　▽　▽　▽　▽　▽　▽

INTRODUCTION

SEE TEXT PAGES

Aortic stenosis occurs when the aortic valve narrows. The left ventricle (LV) has to work harder to move blood through the narrowed opening. If left untreated, the ultimate outcome of this disorder is heart failure.

SUPPORTING ASSESSMENT DATA

▼
▼
▼
▼
▼
▼
▼
▼
▼

If your assessment findings are similar to those listed here, they may suggest aortic stenosis.

▲ Health History:

In addition to the health risk factors listed in Chapter 7, "Coronary Artery Disease," consider at risk patients to whom the following conditions apply:
- History of angina
- Between ages 50 and 70
- Men (80% of victims)
- Family or personal history of congenital aortic bicuspid valve
- Family or personal history of congenital stenosis of pulmonary valve cusps
- History of rheumatic fever
- History of hypertension
- Elderly and atherosclerotic

▲ Physical Findings:

Patients with aortic stenosis complain of the following:
- Angina
- Syncope with exertion
- Fatigue and weakness
- Dyspnea
- Orthopnea

If the patient is in LV failure, he or she will have the complaints listed in Physical Findings of Chapter 12, "Congestive Heart Failure and Pulmonary Edema."

NURSE ALERT:

Patients may be asymptomatic.

AMBULATORY CARE

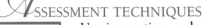

When you assess an ambulatory patient with known aortic stenosis, ask these questions:
- Do you wear medical alert identification?
- Do you take digoxin or warfarin?
- Have you ever had aortic valve replacement, valvuloplasty, or commissurotomy?

ASSESSMENT TECHNIQUES

Use inspection, palpation, and auscultation to assess the patient.

The following symptoms may be evident upon inspection:
- Anxiety
- Difficulty breathing
- Compromised mental status
- Cyanosis
- Peripheral edema
- Hair loss
- Shiny skin over shins

The following symptoms may be evident upon palpation:
- Forceful, sustained apical impulse
- Delayed carotid upstroke
- Cool extremities
- Pulsus alterans
- Decreased systolic blood pressure
- Inferiorly and laterally displaced apex
- Systolic thrill in aortic area at jugular notch and along carotid arteries
- Pulmonary edema
- Narrowed pulse pressure

NURSE ALERT:
You may have to check for systolic thrill while the patient exhales and leans forward.

The following symptoms may be evident upon auscultation:
- S_3 or S_4
- Grade 3 or 4 systolic ejection murmur (especially with children and adolescents with noncalcified valves); not present with calcified valve
- Crescendo-decrescendo murmur heard in aortic area— radiates up neck
- Split S_2

Other findings include palpitations.

DIAGNOSTIC TEST FINDINGS

TEST	FINDINGS
Chest X-ray	• Cardiac enlargement (advanced stenosis) • LV hypertrophy • Pulmonary vein congestion • Aortic valve calcification
12-Lead ECG	• LA hypertrophy (advanced stenosis) • LV hypertrophy (advanced stenosis) • Strain pattern • Left axis deviation • Conduction defects • Atrial fibrillation (advanced stenosis)
Echocardiography	• Aortic valve shows decreased or absent movement • LA enlargement • LV hypertrophy • Abnormal valve orifice
Cardiac catheterization	• Elevated LV systolic pressure • Elevated LV end-diastolic pressure • LV/aorta pressure gradient >50 mm Hg • Elevated LA pressure • Compromised aortic valve area - location of obstruction - Mild stenosis = 1.0 to 1.2 cm - Moderate stenosis = 0.7 to 1 cm - Severe stenosis = <0.5 cm
Radionuclide studies	• Abnormal LV function • Abnormal ejection fraction

PATHOPHYSIOLOGY

Aortic stenosis can be congenital or acquired, resulting from adhesions and fusion of the valve cusps. The following flowchart illustrates its pathophysiology.

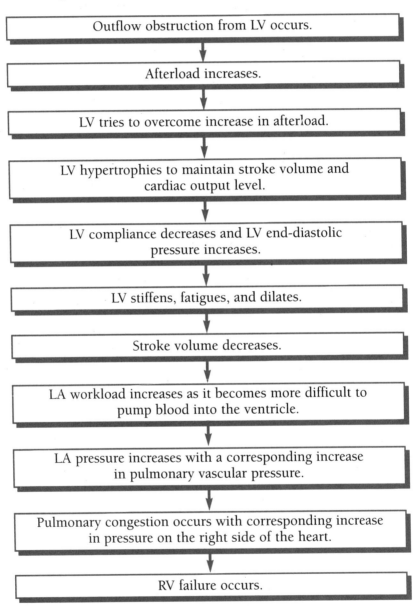

Chapter 16. Aortic Insufficiency

▽ ▽ ▽ ▽ ▽ ▽ ▽

INTRODUCTION

SEE TEXT PAGES

Aortic insufficiency occurs when the aortic valve cannot close during diastole, thereby causing regurgitation.

SUPPORTING ASSESSMENT DATA

If your assessment findings are similar to those listed here, they may suggest aortic insufficiency.

▲ Health History:

In addition to the health risk factors listed in Chapter 7, "Coronary Artery Disease," consider at risk patients who have a history of the following:
- Congenital malformation (personal or familial)
- Idiopathic calcification of the aortic valve
- Rheumatic fever
- Endocarditis, either fungal or bacterial
- Rheumatic spondylitis
- Ehlers-Danlos syndrome
- Lupus erythematosus
- Syphilis
- Aortic dissection
- Rupture of sinus of Valsalva aneurysm
- Hypertension
- Marfan's syndrome

▲ Physical Findings:

Patients with aortic stenosis complain of the following:
- Decreasing blood pressure
- Palpitations, forceful heartbeat
- Syncope on exertion
- Fatigue and weakness
- Dyspnea
- Orthopnea

If the patient is in left-ventricular (LV) failure, he or she will have the complaints listed in Physical Findings of Chapter 12, "Congestive Heart Failure and Pulmonary Edema."

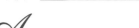

AMBULATORY CARE

When you assess the ambulatory patient with aortic insufficiency, ask these questions:

- Do you wear medical alert identification?
- Have you ever had an aortic valve replacement?
- Do you take warfarin?

ASSESSMENT TECHNIQUES

Use inspection, palpation, percussion, and auscultation to assess the patient.

You may discover the following symptoms upon inspection:

- Anxiety
- Compromised mental status
- All the symptoms of LV failure listed in Chapter 12, "Congestive Heart Failure and Pulmonary Edema"
- Peripheral edema
- de Musset's sign (nodding head)
- Flushed skin

You may discover the following symptoms upon palpation:

- Forceful, diffuse apical impulse
- Widened aortic pulse pressure
- Abrupt rise and fall of carotid and other peripheral pulses
- Water-hammer pulse (bounding)
- Quincke's sign (when you press the patient's fingertip, capillaries in nail base pulsate)
- Hill's sign (popliteal blood pressure is about 40 mm Hg greater than brachial blood pressure)

NURSE ALERT:
You may have to check for Hill's sign while the patient exhales and leans forward.

You may discover lateral displacement of cardiac border (cardiomegaly) upon percussion.

You may discover the following symptoms upon auscultation:

- S_3 or S_4
- Grades 1 to 4, high-pitched, blowing, decrescendo systolic murmur in aortic area

DIAGNOSTIC TEST FINDINGS

TEST	FINDINGS
Chest X-ray	• LV hypertrophy • Pulmonary vascular redistribution • Interstitial pulmonary edema • Aortic valve calcification
12-Lead ECG	• Nonspecific ST-segment changes • LA hypertrophy • LV hypertrophy • Sinus tachycardia
Echocardiography	• LV cavity dilation (chronic insufficiency) • Aortic valve abnormalities • Damaged cusps • Vegetative growth on valve leaflets
Cardiac catheterization	• Elevated pulmonary capillary wedge pressure • Elevated LV end-diastolic pressure • Lowered LV systolic pressure • Elevated LA pressure • Elevated right side heart pressure (advanced insufficiency) • Low systemic diastolic pressures • Define amount of insufficiency
Radionuclide studies	• Define amount of regurgitation

𝒫ATHOPHYSIOLOGY

Aortic insufficiency is usually caused by rheumatic fever. The valve cusps may rupture. They may develop vegetations. They may be perforated with scarring, degeneration, or prolapse, or the valve may become fibrotic. Whatever the cause, the valve tissues retract and the valve cannot close during diastole. As a result, the valve allows backward flow, with corresponding damage to the heart. The following flowchart illustrates the pathophysiology of this disorder.

AORTIC INSUFFICIENCY

Aortic valve becomes incompetent
(cusps become fibrotic and retract).

↓

Blood from the aorta regurgitates to the LV during diastole.

↓

In chronic aortic insufficiency, the LV attempts to compensate
for regurgitation by increasing its forward stroke.

↓

The LV dilates and hypertrophies.

↓

In acute aortic insufficiency, regurgitation causes volume
overload and the LV end-diastolic pressure elevates.

↓

Low aortic diastolic pressures also reduce blood flow
to coronary arteries during diastole.

↓

If undiagnosed or untreated, LV failure occurs.

*S*UGGESTED READINGS

Anderson, H. S., and R. B. Devereux. "Mitral Valve
Prolapse: Guidelines for Diagnosis and Management."
Journal of Musculoskeletal Medicine 11 (January 1994):
38–40, 44–48, 50.

Fisher, J. "Mitral Stenosis: Manifestations and
Management." *Hospital Medicine* 27 (February 1991):
43–53.

Pemerton, A. T. "Update for Nurse Anesthetists—
Anesthetic Techniques for Patients with Valvular Heart
Disease Presenting for Noncardiac Procedures." *AANA
Journal* 61, no. 3 (1993): 314–324.

Rebeyka, D. M. "Caring for a Marfan Patient with
Cardiovascular Complications." *Progress in Cardiovascular
Nursing* 7 (July-September 1992): 6–14.

SECTION V. RELATED VASCULAR DISORDERS

Chapter 17. Aneurysms: Abdominal, Thoracic, and Femoral

▽   ▽   ▽   ▽   ▽   ▽   ▽

INTRODUCTION

SEE TEXT PAGES

An aneurysm occurs when a dilation or bulge appears in the arterial wall.

SUPPORTING ASSESSMENT DATA

If your assessment findings are similar to those listed here, they may suggest the presence of an aneurysm.

▲ Health History:
Consider at risk patients who have a history of the following:
- Arteriosclorosis or atherosclerosis (95%)
- Cystic medial necrosis
- Congenital weakness in artery wall
- Marfan's syndrome
- Hypertension
- Pregnancy
- Peripheral vascular reconstructive surgery
- Trauma or injury
- Syphilis
- Infectious arteritis

▲ Physical Findings:
White men between ages 50 and 80 are most likely to develop abdominal aneurysms. Patients with abdominal aneurysms are likely to have the following:
- No symptoms
- Chronic, severe abdominal pain
- Low back pain unrelated to movement
- Sudden, severe abdominal pain radiating to flank and groin (indicates imminent rupture)
- Pulsation in abdomen
- Nausea and vomiting
- Syncope

- Severe, unrelenting abdominal and back pain similar to renal or ureteral colic (rupture into peritoneal cavity)
- GI bleeding, hematemesis, melena (rupture into duodenum)

▲ Diagnostic Tests:

Abdominal aneurysm is often found on a routine X-ray or during a physical examination. The following tests are useful in diagnosing an abdominal aneurysm:

- Abdominal ultrasound
- Echocardiography
- Anteroposterior and lateral X-ray and computed tomography (CT) to identify the size, shape, and location of the aneurysm.
- A chest X-ray may also show aortic calcification in 75% of patients.

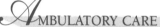 **AMBULATORY CARE**

When assessing the ambulatory patient with an aneurysm, ask these questions:

- Have you ever had an aneurysm repair? If so, was a Dacron graft used?
- Do you know how large your aneurysm is?

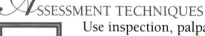 **ASSESSMENT TECHNIQUES**

 Use inspection, palpation, and auscultation to assess the patient. You may discover the following upon inspection:

- Patient asymptomatic
- A thin person that has a pulsating mass in periumbilical area
- For a ruptured aneurysm—pallor, clammy, shock-like symptoms

You may discover the following symptoms upon palpation:
- Tenderness over aneurysm
- Pulsating mass

You may discover the following symptoms upon auscultation:
- Systolic bruit over aorta
- Hypotension (with rupture)

 NURSE ALERT:
Avoid deep palpation because it can cause a rupture.

LOCATION AND SYMPTOMS OF THORACIC AORTIC ANEURYSMS

Thoracic aortic aneurysms most often occur in men over age 60. Patients with thoracic aortic aneurysms are likely to have the following symptoms.

LOCATION	SYMPTOMS
Transverse	• Asymptomatic in early stages • Hoarseness • Throat pain • Dysphagia • Dry cough • Pain radiating to neck, shoulders, lower back, abdomen • GI bleeding, hematemesis, melena (rupture into duodenum)
Dissecting ascending aneurysm	• Ripping sensation in thorax or right anterior chest • Intense onset **NURSE ALERT:** This type of aneurysm is often confused with myocardial infarction (MI).
Dissecting descending aneurysm	• Cyanosis • Leg weakness • Transient paralysis of leg • Neurologic deficits

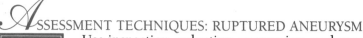

ASSESSMENT TECHNIQUES: RUPTURED ANEURYSM

Use inspection, palpation, percussion, and auscultation to assess the patient. You may discover the following symptoms upon inspection in a patient with a ruptured aneurysm:
- Pallor
- Cyanosis
- Dyspnea
- Diaphoresis

You may discover diminished or absent radial and femoral pulse in the right and left carotid arteries (dissecting ascending aneurysm) upon palpation.

You may discover dullness over the heart upon percussion.

You may discover the following symptoms upon auscultation:
- Aortic insufficiency murmur, diastolic murmur, pericardial friction rub, normal to high blood pressure, substantial asymmetry in pressure between right and left arm (dissecting ascending aneurysm)
- Bilateral crackles and rhonchi, normal blood pressure (dissecting descending aneurysm)

DIAGNOSTIC TESTS

Thoracic aortic aneurysm is usually found on a routine chest X-ray. The following tests are also useful diagnostic tools.

TEST	FINDINGS
Aortography	Location and size of aneurysm
Magnetic resonance imaging	Location of aortic dissection
CT scan	Location of aortic dissection
ECG	Rules out MI
Echocardiography	Presence of dissecting aneurysm in aortic root
Hemoglobin level	Low with leaking aneurysm

FEMORAL AND POPLITEAL ANEURYSMS: SIGNS AND SYMPTOMS

Femoral and popliteal aneurysms are also called peripheral arterial aneurysms. They can be shaped like a spindle (fusiform), which is the most common type, or like a pouch (saccular).

Patients with femoral and popliteal aneurysms are likely to have the following symptoms:
• Pain in the popliteal space
• Edema and venous distention
• Ischemia in the leg or foot
• Severe pain in the leg or foot

Use inspection and palpation to assess the patient. You may discover the following symptoms upon inspection:
• Pallor in leg or foot
• Edema
• Distended veins
• Gangrene

You may discover the following symptoms upon palpation:
• Coldness in the leg or foot
• Loss of pulse
• Pulsating mass
• Firm mass (thrombosis present)

PATHOPHYSIOLOGY

To confirm the diagnosis of aneurysm, a 50% increase in vessel size at the site must occur. Most aneurysms are caused by congenitally low elastin. Whatever the trigger may be, degenerative changes cause weakness in the muscle wall. The vessel bulges at this spot; the wall continues to weaken, and the aneurysm enlarges and eventually ruptures.

Because the aorta is large, it experiences more stress than any other part of the arterial system. Four times as many aneurysms occur in the abdominal aorta as anywhere else. After an abdominal aneurysm has reached 6 cm, there is a 20% chance that it will rupture during the next 12 months. Fifty percent of patients with ruptured abdominal aneurysms die within 2 years; 85% die within 5 years.

Chapter 18. Atherosclerotic Arterial Occlusive Disease

▽　▽　▽　▽　▽　▽　▽

INTRODUCTION

SEE TEXT PAGES

Atherosclerotic arterial occlusive disease appears when the lumen of the aorta and its major branches suffer an obstruction or narrowing. It usually appears in the lower extremities of men age 50 or older. Many patients who have this condition also have coronary artery disease. See Chapter 7, "Coronary Artery Disease," for assessment guidelines.

NURSE ALERT:
A variant of this disorder, Raynaud's disease, more often afflicts younger patients and women. It is of unknown etiology. Its symptoms include vasospasm in the extremities in response to cold and stress.

SUPPORTING ASSESSMENT DATA

If your assessment findings are similar to those listed here, they may suggest atherosclerotic arterial occlusive disease.

▲ Health History:
In addition to the health risk factors listed in Chapter 7, "Coronary Artery Disease," consider at risk the following patients:
- Men over age 50
- Smokers
- Diabetics

▲ Physical Findings:
Patients with atherosclerotic arterial occlusive disease complain of the following symptoms, which are related to the vessels involved:
- Intermittent claudication (severe pain and cramps in the area of the occlusion after exercise relieved by rest)
- Visual disturbances
- Vertigo
- Headache
- Abdominal pain
- Diarrhea

Ambulatory Care

When you assess the ambulatory patient, ask these questions:

- Are you taking any blood pressure, heart, or diabetes medications?
- How far can you walk without pain?
- Have you ever taken pentoxfylline?
- Do you take aspirin daily?
- Do you take any medication for pain? How often?
- Have you ever had an embolectomy, endarterectomy, angioplasty or laser surgery, or bypass grafting in the extremities?
- Have you ever had an exercise (or nonexercise, dipyridamole) stress test?
- Are you taking any beta blocker medication?

NURSE ALERT:
Beta blockers have peripheral vasoconstricting effects. Patients with atherosclerotic arterial occlusive disease should not take beta blockers.

Assessment Techniques

Use inspection, palpation, and auscultation to assess the patient.

You may discover the following symptoms upon inspection:

- Leg ulcers
- Gangrene
- Shiny skin
- Thickened or deformed nails
- Loss of hair in affected area
- Pallor in area affected by occlusion
- Areas of decreased circulation
- Bluish extremities

You may discover the following symptoms upon palpation:

- Decreased sensory or motor function in affected area
- Decreased pulse amplitude distal to occlusion
- Increased amplitude of peripheral pulses
- Capillary filling in 3 seconds or more (normal is less than or equal to 3 seconds)
- Cool skin

You may discover upon auscultation audible bruits over occluded vessels.

DIAGNOSTIC TESTS

TEST	FINDINGS
Angiography	• Location of obstruction • Vascular lesions
Duplex imaging (ultrasonography)	• Plaque formation • Abnormal flow and pressure
Doppler flow studies	• Abnormal blood flow through arteries indicated by low-pitched sound and monophasic waveform
Exercise testing	• Precipitates ischemia and claudication
Digital subtraction angiography	• Occlusion
Oscillometry	• Occlusive sites
Electroencephalography and computed tomography	• Brain lesions

ᏢATHOPHYSIOLOGY

Atherosclerotic arterial occlusive disease involves changes in the affected artery, including accumulation of lipids, carbohydrates, calcium, blood components, and fibrous tissue. The lumen of the vessel narrows, thus reducing blood flow. Although it's a different process than arteriosclerosis, the two often occur at the same time.

At times, a blood clot causes obstruction. The clot may form in response to an injury or fracture, or it may be the result of emboli, thrombosis, or plaque. It can affect the internal and external carotid, vertebral and basilar, innominate (brachiocephalic), subclavian, mesenteric, femoral, popliteal, and iliac arteries. An aneurysm can also occur. Survival of tissue depends on rapid diagnosis and removal of the obstruction.

*C*hapter 19. Arterial Embolism

▽ ▽ ▽ ▽ ▽ ▽ ▽

*I*NTRODUCTION

SEE TEXT PAGES

An arterial embolism is an obstruction of blood flow through a vessel caused by a fragment traveling in the arterial circulation. It results in tissue hypoxia and cellular death.

*S*UPPORTING ASSESSMENT DATA

▼
▼
▼
▼
▼
▼
▼
▼
▼
▼

If your assessment findings are similar to those listed here, they may suggest arterial embolism.

▲ Health History:
In addition to the health risk factors listed in Chapter 7, "Coronary Artery Disease," consider at risk patients with a history of the following:
- Vascular injury
- Vascular surgery
- Infections like cellulitis
- Valvular heart disease
- Cardiac arrhythmias
- Myocardial infarction
- Atherosclerosis
- Ventricular aneurysm

▲ Physical Findings:
In addition to the symptoms described in Chapter 18, "Atherosclerotic Arterial Occlusive Disease," patients with arterial embolism complain of the following:
- Sudden, severe pain
- Gradual loss of sensory and motor functioning within 18 hours of occlusion

*A*SSESSMENT TECHNIQUES

Use inspection, palpation, and auscultation to assess the patient.

In addition to the findings listed under Assessment Techniques in Chapter 18, "Atherosclerotic Arterial Occlusive Disease," you may discover darkened or mottled extremities upon inspection.

Findings upon palpation are the same as those described under Assessment Techniques in Chapter 18, "Atherosclerotic Arterial Occlusive Disease."

Findings upon auscultation are the same as those described under Assessment Techniques in Chapter 18, "Atherosclerotic Arterial Occlusive Disease."

DIAGNOSTIC TESTS

TEST	FINDINGS
Angiography	• Location of embolus
Doppler flow studies	• Abnormal (decreased or absent) blood flow distal to embolus

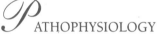

PATHOPHYSIOLOGY

An embolism can be caused by a fragment of thrombus, fat, tissue, or atherosclerotic lesion. It can also be caused by bacteria or an air bubble.

Usually, an embolism is caused by a fragment of thrombus that originates in the chambers of the heart. This process follows valvular heart disease, atrial fibrillation, myocardial infarction, congestive heart failure, vascular injury, or an infection.

Once the obstruction occurs, tissue damage varies according to embolus size, location, degree of obstruction, and involvement of distal tissue.

Chapter 20. Venous Thrombosis and Thrombophlebitis

▽ ▽ ▽ ▽ ▽ ▽ ▽

INTRODUCTION

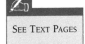

SEE TEXT PAGES

Venous thrombosis and venous thrombophlebitis occur when a venous thrombus develops and is followed by inflammation. While these are actually two different conditions, in practice they are treated similarly.

SUPPORTING ASSESSMENT DATA

If your assessment findings are similar to those listed here, they may suggest venous thrombosis or thrombophlebitis.

▲ Health History:

In addition to the health risk factors listed in Chapter 7, "Coronary Artery Disease," consider at risk patients with a history of the following:

- Prolonged bed rest
- Recent leg trauma
- Venous access with irritating solutions
- Liver disease
- Withdraw from anticoagulant therapy
- Recent surgery
- Recent or current oral contraceptive use
- Obesity
- Congestive heart failure
- Recently had anesthesia
- Recently been in shock
- Varicose veins (see Chapter 21, "Varicose Veins," for a discussion of this condition)

▲ Physical Findings:

Patients with this condition complain of pain and tenderness.

AMBULATORY CARE

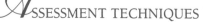

When you assess an ambulatory patient, ask these questions:
- Have you ever had a pulmonary embolus?
- Have you ever taken Coumadin?
- Have you ever had a thrombectomy or had a Greenfield filter placed in your leg?

ASSESSMENT TECHNIQUES

Use inspection and palpation to assess the patient.

You may discover the following symptoms upon inspection:
- Unilateral leg swelling
- Localized warmth (inflammation)
- Prominent superficial veins

You may discover the following symptoms upon palpation:
- Knot or bump in the region of the thrombus
- Redness and swelling at the site
- Pain on dorsiflexion of the foot (Homans' sign)

NURSE ALERT:
The first sign of this disorder may be pulmonary embolism. If you suspect pulmonary embolism, never test for Homans' sign. The test can cause another embolism.

DIAGNOSTIC TESTS

TEST	FINDINGS
Venography (contrast phlebography)	• Absence of filling
Doppler flow ultrasonography	• Changes in blood flow secondary to thrombus

DIAGNOSTIC TESTS (*CONTINUED*)

TEST	FINDINGS
Duplex imaging ultrasonography	• Abnormal flow and pressure in afflicted vein
I-fibrinogen injection	• Formation of clots
Impedance plethysmography	• Abnormal blood flow

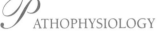

ATHOPHYSIOLOGY

Disorders of the venous system, including venous stasis, hemoconcentration, venous trauma, inflammation, and altered coagulation, contribute to the formation of thrombi. This is a serious condition that can result in embolization.

Chapter 21. Varicose Veins

▽ ▽ ▽ ▽ ▽ ▽ ▽

INTRODUCTION

SEE TEXT PAGES

A vein is diagnosed as varicosed if it is enlarged, dilated, and tortuous.

SUPPORTING ASSESSMENT DATA

If your assessment findings are similar to those listed here, they may suggest the presence of varicose veins.

▲ Health History:

Consider at risk patients to whom the following conditions apply:
• Pregnancy (especially having had many pregnancies)
• Over age 50
• Female
• Stand for long periods
• Family history of varicose veins
• Traumatic injury
• History of arterial embolism or vascular thrombosis
• Do not exercise
• Obesity

▲ Physical Findings:

Patients with varicose veins complain of the following symptoms, which may be relieved by exercise:
• Mild to severe aching in legs
• Heaviness, worse at night or in hot weather
• Leg cramps at night
• Aching during menses
• Itching
• Fatigue
• Dilated, tortuous skin veins

AMBULATORY CARE

When you assess an ambulatory patient with varicose veins, ask these questions:
• Have you ever worn support or antiembolism stockings?
• Have you ever had an embolism? Vascular thrombosis?
• Have you ever had vein ligation and stripping?
• Have you ever had sclerotherapy?
• Do you wear tight knee-high stockings or socks or long girdles?

ASSESSMENT TECHNIQUES

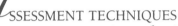

Use inspection, palpation, and auscultation to assess the patient.

You may discover the following symptoms upon inspection:
• Dilated, purplish, rope-like leg veins
• Redness or brown discoloration especially at ankles
• Leg ulcers
• Edema of calves and ankles

You may discover the following symptoms upon palpation:
• Nodules in affected veins
• Tenderness in affected area
• Overly firm calf muscles
• Valve incompetence (manual compression and Trendelenburg's test—see below)

You may discover audible bruits over occluded vessels upon auscultation.

DIAGNOSTIC TESTS

TEST	FINDINGS
Trendelenburg's test • Have the patient stand. • Use a pen to mark vein. • Have the patient lie down and elevate legs for 1 minute. • Have the patient stand, and measure venous filling time.	• Veins with competent valves fill in less than 30 seconds. • If veins again fill in less than 30 seconds, probable incompetent perforating vein and deep vein valves.

DIAGNOSTIC TESTS (CONTINUED)

TEST	FINDINGS
Trendelenburg's test (*continued*) • Have the patient lie down and elevate legs for 1 minute. • Apply a tourniquet to upper thigh. • Have the patient stand, and measure venous filling time. • Remove the tourniquet. • May be repeated with tourniquet just below the knee and then with it around the upper calf.	• If the veins fill in less than 30 seconds, probable incompetent superficial vein valves allowing backward blood flow
Manual compression • Use one hand to palpate distended vein. • Use other hand to compress vein 8 in. (20.3 cm) above the palpation point. • Feel for an impulse with the palpating hand.	• No impulse (competent valves) • Palpable impulse—incompetent valves in vein
Doppler flow ultrasonography	Venous backflow through incompetent valves
Photoplethysmography	Abnormal changes in skin circulation
Phlebography	• Dilation • Incompetent valves • Thrombi
Venous outflow and reflux plethysmography	Deep vein occlusion
Ascending and descending venography (this test is invasive and rarely used)	• Occlusive sites • Patterns of collateral flow

PATHOPHYSIOLOGY

Valvular incompetence and constantly elevated venous pressure cause varicose veins. These two factors cause the classic dilated, tortuous appearance of the vein. Varicose veins often appear in the calves and ankles.

Primary varicose veins afflict patients with an inherited disorder that robs superficial vein walls of elasticity. Pregnancy, standing for long periods, and constrictive clothes can precipitate the disorder. Women are twice as likely to develop primary varicose veins as men. Usually, the disorder affects both legs.

Secondary varicose veins afflict patients who have experienced an injury, a vein obstruction, thrombosis, or inflammation. Such patients have a disorder of the venous system, such as occlusion, that precipitates secondary varicose veins. Such disorders damage the valve of a deep and perforated vein, causing it to become incompetent. Usually, the disorder affects only one leg.

COMPLICATIONS

Varicose veins can ultimately lead to venous insufficiency and ulcers. You will usually find ulcers near or on the ankles of your patient. Abnormal venous pressure ruptures small skin veins and venules. The ulcer then forms.

SUGGESTED READINGS

"Aortic Aneurysm." *Mayo Clinic Newsletter* 12 (March 1994): 7.

Birnbaumer, D. M. "Abdominal Emergencies in Later Life." *Emergency Medicine* 25 (April 1993): 74–82.

Bright, L. D., and S. Georgi. "Peripheral Vascular Disease: Is It Arterial or Venous?" *AJN* 92 (September 1992): 34–47.

Halfman, M., and D. E. Berg. "Venous Thrombosis: Antithrombin III Deficiency." *Critical Care Nursing Clinics of North America* 5 (September 1993): 499–509.

Shaw, E."Screening to Save Lives: The Gloucestershire Aneurysm Screening Project." *Professional Nurse* 8 (December 1992): 185–188.

Stein, P. D., et al. "Strategy for Diagnosis of Patients with Suspected Acute Pulmonary Embolism." *Chest: The Cardiopulmonary Journal* 103 (May 1993): 1533–1599.

SECTION VI: INFLAMMATORY HEART DISEASE

Chapter 22. Pericarditis

▽ ▽ ▽ ▽ ▽ ▽ ▽

INTRODUCTION

SEE TEXT PAGES

Pericarditis is an inflammation of the pericardium. Acute pericarditis can lead to pericardial effusion. If edema occurs too rapidly, the patient may develop cardiac tamponade, which can be fatal.

SUPPORTING ASSESSMENT DATA

If your assessment findings are similar to those listed here, they may suggest pericarditis.

▲ **Health History:**

Consider at risk patients who have a history of the following:
• Bacterial, viral, protozoal, tubercular, or fungal infection
• Neoplasms
• High-dose radiation to the thorax
• Uremia
• Rheumatic fever
• Lupus erythematosus
• Rheumatoid arthritis or other autoimmune disease
• Myocardial infarction (MI; Dressler's syndrome) or other postcardiac injury
• Other injury
• Drug therapy with penicillin, procainamide, hydralazine, corticosteroids, phenytoin, daunorubicin, phenylbutazone, minoxidil
• Myxedema (rare)
• Aortic aneurysm (rare)

▲ **Physical Findings:**

Patients with pericarditis are likely to complain of the following symptoms:
• Severe, sudden pain beginning in the sternum and spreading to the neck, shoulders, back, and arms
• Pain that worsens with a deep breath, moving, or sitting
• Pain that eases on leaning forward

- Pain similar to that of MI
- Chest feels full
- Fever
- Joint pain
- Cough (severe pericarditis)
- Orthopnea
- Fatigue

NURSE ALERT:

If the patient has tuberculosis, has had radiation treatment, or suffers from neoplasms or uremia, he or she may be asymptomatic.

ASSESSMENT TECHNIQUES

Use inspection, palpation, and auscultation to assess the patient.

You may discover the following symptoms upon inspection:
- Anorexia
- Edema (with constrictive pericarditis)
- Symptoms similar to those of right ventricular failure (with constrictive pericarditis)
- Distended neck veins (cardiac tamponade)
- Hepatic congestion
- Restlessness
- Pulsus paradoxus (cardiac tamponade)
- Kussmaul's sign (constrictive pericarditis)
- Dyspnea (cardiac tamponade)
- Pallor (cardiac tamponade)

You may discover the following symptoms upon palpation:
- Diminished or absent apical pulse
- Ascites
- Tachycardia
- Fever
- Hepatojugular reflex
- Clammy skin (cardiac tamponade)
- Hypotension (cardiac tamponade)

You may discover the following symptoms upon auscultation:
- Pericardial friction rub (indicative of pericarditis)
- Distant heart sounds
- S_3 (congestive heart failure)
- Murmurs (valvular dysfunction)
- Narrowed pulse pressure

DIAGNOSTIC TESTS

The following table lists findings in a cluster of diagnostic tests that support a diagnosis of pericarditis. These tests can also indicate the cause of the patient's pericarditis.

TEST	FINDINGS	ETIOLOGY
White blood cell count	Elevated	Infection **NURSE ALERT:** A normal count does not rule out pericarditis.
Erythrocyte sedimentation rate	Elevated	Infection
Serum creatine kinase-MB levels	Elevated	Epicardial inflammation
Cardiac isoenzymes	Elevated	MI
Antinuclear antibodies	Positive	Connective tissue disease
Pericardial fluid culture	Presence of bacteria or fungus	Infection
Blood urea nitrogen levels	Elevated	Uremia
Antistreptolysin-O titer	Elevated	Rheumatic fever
Purified protein derivative skin test	Positive	Tuberculosis

DIAGNOSTIC TESTS (CONTINUED)

TEST	FINDINGS	ETIOLOGY
ECG	• Elevated ST segments in two or three limb leads • Elevated ST segments in precordial leads • No changes in QRS complex morphology • ST-segment depression in V_1 and aVR • Inverted T wave after isoelectric ST segment • Atrial ectopic rhythms • Diminished QRS complex voltage	Pericardial inflammation or effusion
Echocardiography	Space between ventricular wall and pericardium is echo-free	Pericardial effusion

PATHOPHYSIOLOGY

Inflammation of the pericardium, the fibrous sac around the heart, can be either acute or chronic. Patients with acute pericarditis have a good prognosis if they do not develop constriction. Chronic pericarditis is more serious because it causes thickening of the pericardium.
Pericarditis appears secondary to other conditions, such as tuberculosis, uremia, myocardial infarction, or trauma. Its progression is diagrammed here.

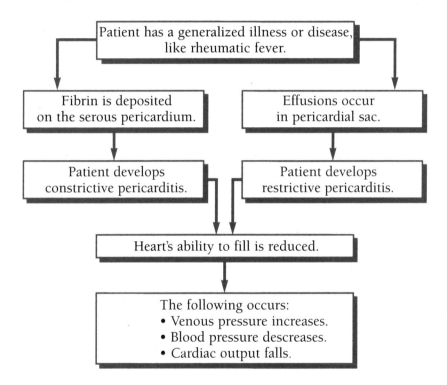

Patient has a generalized illness or disease, like rheumatic fever.

Fibrin is deposited on the serous pericardium.

Effusions occur in pericardial sac.

Patient develops constrictive pericarditis.

Patient develops restrictive pericarditis.

Heart's ability to fill is reduced.

The following occurs:
• Venous pressure increases.
• Blood pressure descreases.
• Cardiac output falls.

*C*hapter 23. Endocarditis

▽   ▽   ▽   ▽   ▽   ▽   ▽

*I*NTRODUCTION

SEE TEXT PAGES

Endocarditis is an infection of the endothelial lining in the heart. Many patients with endocarditis (40%) do not have any other heart disease.

*S*UPPORTING ASSESSMENT DATA

If your assessment findings are similar to those listed here, they may suggest endocarditis.

▲ Health History:

Consider at risk, patients who have a history of:
- Recent open heart surgery with artificial valve replacement
- Recent invasive procedures of any kind (gynecologic, dental)
- Rheumatic valvular disease
- Mitral valve prolapse
- Degenerative heart disease
- Calcific aortic stenosis (elderly patients)
- Valvular lesions
- Weight loss
- Cardiac lesions
- Septic thrombophlebitis
- I.V. drug use
- Immunosuppressant therapy
- Any infection (usual cause—*Streptococcus viridans*)
- Marfan's syndrome
- Skin abscess
- Bone infection
- Pulmonary infection

When you assess a patient for endocarditis, get a complete description of his or her existing symptoms or illness. Determine if your patient has a history of any of the risk factors listed above.

▲ Physical Findings:

Patients with endocarditis are likely to complain of the following symptoms:

- Pain in the upper left chest and shoulder (splenic infarction)
- Flank pain (renal infarction)
- Sudden pain in chest or shoulder
- Joint pain
- Anorexia
- Pain similar to that of MI
- Dyspnea
- Cough
- Fever
- Chills
- Nausea and vomiting
- Numbness or tingling in extremities
- Myalgia
- Disruption or loss of vision
- Exercise intolerance (congestive heart failure [CHF])
- Diaphoresis
- Fatigue

ASSESSMENT TECHNIQUES

In addition to exploring risk factors and patient complaints, use inspection, percussion, palpation, and auscultation to assess your patient.

You may discover the following symptoms upon inspection:
- Splinter hemorrhaging under nails
- Edema
- Anorexia
- Cough with bloody phlegm (pulmonary infection secondary to right side endocarditis)
- Diaphoresis
- Petechiae (skin on trunk and buccal, pharyngeal, and conjunctival mucosa)
- Nodes on fingers (Osler's nodes—rare)
- Retinal hemorrhages with white centers (Roth's spots)
- Signs of peripheral gangrene
- Purple lesions on palms and soles (Janeway lesions)
- Inflamed, pustular lesions on skin
- Clubbed fingers (advanced endocarditis)
- Any symptoms of heart failure
- CNS symptoms such as headache, confusion, and aphasia (brain embolism)
- Signs of glomerulonephritis (allergic, immunologic)
- Dyspnea (lung infarction)
- Tachycardia
- Pallor
- Tachypnea (lung infarction)

- Hemoptysis (lung infarction)
- Cyanosis (lung infarction)
- Hematuria (kidney infarction)

You may discover dullness in the lower sternum (**enlarged spleen**) upon percussion.

You may discover the following symptoms upon **palpation:**
- Diminished or absent pulse in any cold limbs due to emboli
- Abdominal pain (mesenteric emboli) or rigidity (**splenic infarction**)
- Enlarged spleen (splenic infarction)
- Diminished renal, peripheral, and cerebral profusion (embolization)
- Thrills (murmurs)
- Hepatojugular reflex (CHF)
- Enlarged liver (CHF)
- Distended neck veins (CHF)
- Peripheral edema (CHF)

You may discover the following symptoms upon **auscultation:**
- Insufficiency and stenosis murmurs in any valve
- Diminished or absent breath sounds (lung infarction)
- Pleural friction rub (pulmonary infection secondary to right side endocarditis)
- Crackles (CHF)

NURSE ALERT:
If you find a sudden change in a murmur or a new murmur and if either is accompanied by fever, suspect **endocarditis** immediately.

DIAGNOSTIC TESTS

The organism that has caused the endocarditis can usually be diagnosed by taking at least three blood cultures in a 24- to 48-hour period. If the blood cultures are negative, the infection could be caused by a fungus or by an organism that is difficult to culture.

In addition to these cultures and any abnormal test results associated with specific organs, such as the lungs or kidneys, you can use the tests listed in the following table to support a diagnosis of endocarditis. These tests can also indicate the cause of the endocarditis.

TEST	FINDINGS	ETIOLOGY
Erythrocyte sedimentation rate	Often elevated	Infection
Serum creatinine	Elevated	Infection
Complete blood count	•Low hemoglobin •Elevated white cell count	Anemia Infection

!

NURSE ALERT: A normal count does not rule out subacute endocarditis.

TEST	FINDINGS	ETIOLOGY
Rheumatoid factor	Elevated	Infection
Immune complex levels	Elevated	Infection
Blood cultures	Positive	Infection
Echocardiography	•Abnormal wall motion •Abnormal valves	CHF

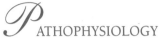

PATHOPHYSIOLOGY

Infection of the endothelial lining of the heart, or endocarditis, is either subacute or acute. It is most likely to involve the left side of the heart. Microbes like *Streptococcus viridans*, which are unlikely to affect other tissue, cause subacute endocarditis. Subacute endocarditis usually takes weeks to months to develop.

Any pathogen that can directly attack tissue can cause acute endocarditis. Acute endocarditis can appear in days or weeks, and it progresses rapidly. When untreated, endocarditis is fatal. When treated, 70% of patients recover. Endocarditis that damages the valves or involves a prosthetic valve has a poor prognosis.

Valvular insufficiency, septal defects, artificial valves, and so on cause trauma to the endothelial lining.

↓

Platelets and fibrin form thrombi.

↓

Nonbacterial endocarditis develops.

↓

Bacteria from infections of skin, kidneys, and so on colonize valves.

↓

Deposits of platelets and fibrin continue to form (usually on left side of heart).

↓

Vegetative growth appears, deforming and destroying damaged valve tissue and normal tissue.

↓

Continuous presence of antigenemia and antibodies results in high immune complex levels.

↓

Peripheral areas, like the kidneys and lungs, become hypersensitive (allergic vasculitis).

↓

Embolization can follow and travel to the heart, kidneys, lungs, and so on.

*C*hapter 24. Myocarditis

▽   ▽   ▽   ▽   ▽   ▽   ▽

*I*NTRODUCTION

SEE TEXT PAGES

Myocarditis is an inflammation of the myocardium. Giant cell myocarditis, which is rare, has no known cause.

*S*UPPORTING ASSESSMENT DATA

▼
▼
▼
▼
▼
▼
▼
▼
▼

If your assessment findings are similar to those listed here, they may suggest myocarditis.

▲ Health History:

Consider at risk patients who have or have had:
• A virus infection, particularly coxsackievirus A and B. Other viruses that may cause this disorder include HIV, adenoviruses, poliomyelitis, influenza, rubeola, rubella, and echoviruses.
• A bacterial infection, including diphtheria, tuberculosis, typhoid, tetanus, and Lyme disease, and staphylococcal, pneumococcal, and gonococcal bacteria
• Rheumatic fever
• Postcardiotomy syndrome
• Radiation therapy
• Alcoholism or other chemical toxicity
• Parasites, particularly toxoplasmosis and trypanosomiasis in infants and adults with autoimmune disorders
• Helminthic infections like trichinosis

▲ Physical Findings:

Patients with myocarditis may complain of the following:
• Fatigue
• Dyspnea
• Palpitations
• Tachycardia
• Mild, non–angina–like chest pressure or pain
• Persistent fever

*A*SSESSMENT TECHNIQUES

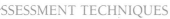

Use inspection, palpation, and auscultation to assess the patient.

You may discover the following symptoms upon inspection:
- Neck vein distention indicative of left ventricular failure. See Chapter 12, "Congestive Heart Failure and Pulmonary Edema," for additional assessment guidelines.
- Difficulty breathing

You may discover tachycardia abnormal for degree of fever upon palpation.

You may discover the following symptoms upon auscultation:
- Mitral insufficiency murmur (rarely)
- Pericardial friction rub (pericarditis)
- Muffled S_1
- Diastolic gallop (S_3)
- Atrial gallop (S_4)

DIAGNOSTIC TESTS

TEST	FINDINGS
Endomyocardial biopsy	• Myocarditis
Cardiac enzyme levels	• Elevated
Complete blood count	• Elevated white blood cell count
Erythrocyte sedimentation rate	• Elevated
Antibody titers	• Elevated (may indicate rheumatic fever; see Chapter 25, "Rheumatic Heart Disease")

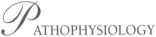

PATHOPHYSIOLOGY

Myocarditis rarely causes long-term problems and usually corrects itself. Your patient may have a chronic (recurring) or acute (one event) myocarditis. On the rare occasions that myocarditis becomes critical, it can cause degeneration of myofibrils, right and left ventricular failure, cardiomyopathy (rare), chronic valvulitis (with rheumatic fever), thromboembolism, and arrhythmias.

$\mathscr{C}$hapter 25. Rheumatic Heart Disease

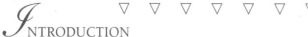

$\mathscr{I}$NTRODUCTION

SEE TEXT PAGES

Rheumatic fever precipitates rheumatic heart disease. (Refer to Section IV on Valvular Heart Disease.) Rheumatic heart disease is a serious condition, particularly if undiagnosed or untreated. Refer to chapters 13 through 16 for specific valvular disease assessments and chapters 22 through 24 for inflammatory consequences of rheumatic fever.

$\mathscr{S}$UPPORTING ASSESSMENT DATA

▼
▼
▼
▼
▼
▼
▼
▼
▼
▼

If your assessment findings are similar to those listed here, they may suggest rheumatic heart disease.

▲ Health History:
Consider at risk, patients who:
• Are children
• Are malnourished or living in crowded conditions
• Have rheumatic fever
• Have had a recent low-grade fever

▲ Physical Findings:
Patients with rheumatic fever are likely to complain of the following symptoms:
• Streptococcal infection in the past 6 weeks
• Low-grade fever that spikes in the late afternoon
• Epistaxis
• Joint pain

$\mathscr{A}$SSESSMENT TECHNIQUES

Use inspection, palpation, and auscultation to assess the patient for rheumatic fever.

You may discover the following symptoms upon inspection:
• Skin lesions, like erythema marginatum, that are red with white centers and defined borders (indicative of carditis)
• Edema

- Mild to severe chorea
- Joint redness

You may discover the following symptoms upon palpation:
- Subcutaneous nodules (3 mm to 2 cm) near tendons or joints (indicative of carditis)
- Rapid pulse

You may discover the following symptoms upon auscultation:
- Pericardial friction rub (indicative of pericarditis)
- Bibasilar crackles and ventricular or atrial gallop (indicative of left ventricular failure)
- A systolic murmur of mitral insufficiency
- A midsystolic murmur (indicative of edema and stiffness in mitral leaflet)
- A diastolic murmur of aortic insufficiency (rare)

DIAGNOSTIC TESTS

There is no definitive laboratory test for rheumatic fever. The following table lists findings in a cluster of tests that support the diagnosis.

TEST	FINDINGS
Erythrocyte sedimentation rate	• Elevated
Complete blood count	• Slight anemia (decreased hemoglobin and hematocrit) • Elevated white blood cell count
C-reactive protein	• Positive, particularly when disease is acute
Cardiac enzyme levels	• Elevated, indicative of severe carditis
Antistreptolysin-O titer	• Elevated within past 2 months in 95% of patients

DIAGNOSTIC TESTS (CONTINUED)

TEST	FINDINGS
Throat culture	• Group A streptococci 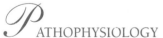 **NURSE ALERT:** Negative results do not rule out streptococcal infection. The bacteria is difficult to isolate and culture.
ECG	• About 20% may show prolonged PR interval
Chest X-ray	• Abnormal (indicative of myocarditis, heart failure, pericardial effusion)
Echocardiography	• Valvular damage • Abnormal chamber size • Impaired left ventricular function • Pericardial effusion
Cardiac catheterization	• Valvular damage • Impaired left ventricular function

𝒫ATHOPHYSIOLOGY

Rheumatic fever, which involves the joints, heart, CNS, and skin and subcutaneous tissues, appears secondary to a group A streptococcal infection. Antibodies specific to streptococcus A organisms begin to react to tissue sites by producing lesions. Because this occurs in only a small percentage of people with this streptococcal infection, victims probably have altered host resistance. Rheumatic fever is a disease of children and adolescents and often recurs.

Rheumatic heart disease is the most serious complication of rheumatic fever. It appears in half of patients with rheumatic fever. The disease can attack the myocardium, endocardium, or pericardium in its early stages. In its later stages, it may attack the heart valves, causing insufficiency or stenosis.

Rheumatic heart disease can leave the heart permanently damaged. Myocarditis can cause nodules and scarring. Endocarditis damages the mitral valve leaflet in females and the aortic valve leaflet in males. It can also damage the tricuspid valve and, rarely, the pulmonary valve.

Early diagnosis and long-term treatment with antibiotics are critical to preventing cardiac and valvular damage.

SUGGESTED READINGS

Christensen, M. A. "Myocardial Contusion: New Concepts in Diagnosis and Management." *American Journal of Critical Care* 2 (1993): 28–34.

Feldman, T. "Rheumatic Mitral Stenosis: On the Rise Again, Part 3." *Postgraduate Medicine* 93 (May 1993): 93–197.

Kontos, C. D., and M. L. Hess. "Today's Approach to Managing Severe Myocarditis." *Journal of Critical Illness* 9 (February 1994): 152–158.

Spodick, D. "Pathogenesis of Edema in Constrictive Pericarditis." *Circulation* 85 (1992): 848.

Steckelberg, J. M., and W. R. Wilson. "Risk Factors for Ineffective Endocarditis." *Infectious Disease Clinics of North America* 7 (March 1993): 9–19.

Chapter 26. Pacemakers

▽ ▽ ▽ ▽ ▽ ▽ ▽

INTRODUCTION

SEE TEXT PAGES

Pacemakers are used to correct cardiac abnormalities. After your patient has a pacemaker inserted, you'll need to assess how well it is working and observe your patient for adverse reactions.

SUPPORTING ASSESSMENT DATA

Pacemaker candidates are likely to have a history of the symptoms listed here.

▲ **Health History:**
• Dizziness
• Exercise intolerance
• Syncope
• Fainting
• An episode of cardiac arrest

Temporary pacemakers are used in ICUs and CCUs. They may be used for tachycardia and pacing the heart after cardiac surgery or preceding the need for a permanent pacemaker.

Patients with permanent pacemakers are likely to have one of the following conditions:
• Recurring conduction block
• Sick sinus syndrome
• Sinus arrest
• Sinoatrial block
• Symptomatic brachycardia
• Adams-Stokes syncope (intermittent heart block)
• Ectopic rhythms precipitated by antiarrhythmic medication
• Tachyarrhythmia that does not respond to treatment

▲ **Physical Findings:**
Patients who are having problems with their pacemakers may complain of the following symptoms after surgery:

- Pain around insertion site
- Excessive or bloody drainage from insertion site
- Redness or warmth around insertion site
- Swelling around insertion site
- Ecchymosis
- Impaired mobility of upper extremities

Later, they may complain of the following:
- Difficulty breathing
- Dizziness
- Pulse below the lower rate limit
- Edema
- Uncontrollable hiccups
- Chest pain
- Fever
- Feeling of fullness in the chest
- Fainting

NURSE ALERT:
Make sure the patient understands that he or she should report any of the above symptoms immediately because they may indicate pacemaker failure.

AMBULATORY CARE

When you assess an ambulatory patient who has a pacemaker, ask these questions:
- Have you ever had a battery replacement?
- Do you carry medical alert identification with your name; your physician's name, address, and phone; and the pacemaker type and settings? (Regularly remind your patient about the importance of this card. He or she should always carry it and show it when travelling by air. Although the pacemaker sets off metal detectors, neither the pacemaker nor the patient is harmed.)
- Do you wear medical alert identification?
- When did you last have your pacemaker checked?
- Do you check your pacemaker at regular intervals?
- What heart medications do you take?

ASSESSMENT TECHNIQUES

You may discover symptoms of one or more of the following conditions when you assess your patient:
- Venous thrombosis
- Embolism
- Infection
- Stimulation of the pectoral, or diaphragmatic muscle
- Pneumothorax
- Arrhythmias
- Cardiac tamponade (caused by perforated ventricle, rare)
- Heart failure
- Abnormal operation of device

PACEMAKER PROBLEMS

PROBLEM	DIAGNOSTIC TOOL	CAUSE
Failure to pace	ECG shows loss of pacemaker spike	• Battery needs to be replaced • Dislodged lead • Fractured lead wire internal to catheter • Catheter is disconnected from generator • Sensing malfunction
Failure to capture	ECG shows pacemaker spike not followed by a QRS or P wave	• Low voltage • Battery needs to be replaced • Catheter is disconnected from generator • Catheter is in wrong position • Fractured catheter or wire • Fibrosis at catheter tip
Failure to sense	ECG shows spikes out of sync with patient's rhythm. This is called pacemaker competition.	• Catheter wire fractured • Catheter tip has moved • Battery failure • Sensitivity setting too low

PACEMAKER JARGON

TERM	MEANING
Artifact	ECG spike corresponding to electrical impulse discharged by the device's generator.
Capture	When the pulse generator discharges, the heart contracts. This is called "capture."
Electrode	The thin conductive wire that is in direct contact with the heart. The electrode continuously sends information about heart function to the pulse generator.
Failure to capture	The heart does not respond to the pacing stimulus.
Failure to pace	No artifact shows up on the ECG when the pacemaker should be firing.
Failure to sense	The pulse generator does not respond to every signal sent by the electrode.
Firing loss	Failure to both sense and capture. The unit has malfunctioned.
Lead	The wire and electrode that receive sensing information from the heart and deliver an impulse to the heart in response to that information.
Oversensing	The pulse generator is too sensitive and responds too quickly to impulse generation signals.
Pulse generator	The power source and circuitry used to sense cardiac activity and send pacing signals.

PACEMAKER JARGON (CONTINUED)

TERM	MEANING
Sensing	The correct recognition of the electrical signals to discharge an impulse or to inhibit discharge.
Threshold	Total electrical energy to maintain continuous depolarization.
Undersensing	The pulse generator periodically fails to respond to the signal from the electrode.

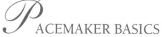ACEMAKER BASICS

The pacemaker is a surgically implanted, battery-powered device that generates a pulse. That pulse stimulates the heart to function normally. Most pacemakers today can be programmed. This feature makes it possible to adjust the device to the patient's need for pacing.

The most common pacemaker is a demand pacemaker. If the patient's heart rate drops below a preset minimum rate, the pacemaker sends an electrical signal to stimulate contraction. Some pacemakers can sense any abnormality in heart rate and either raise or lower the heart rate, whichever is required.

Pacemaker Codes

Because there are so many different kinds of pacemakers, the international group North American Society for Pacing and Electrophysiology/British Electrophysiology Group (NASPE/BPEG) has established a five-letter coding system. Pacemakers are classified according to this five-letter code.

The first letter indicates the paced chamber. There are five possibilities:
• V - Ventricle
• A - Atrium
• D - Dual
• S - Single Chamber
• O - None

The second letter indicates the sensed chamber. There are five possibilities:
- V - Ventricle
- A - Atrium
- D - Dual
- S - Single Chamber
- O - None

The third letter indicates the mode of response to sensing. There are four possibilities:
- T - Triggered by ventricular activity
- I - Inhibited by ventricular activity
- D - Dual (atrial triggered, ventricular inhibited)
- O - Neither (continuous)

The fourth letter indicates any programmable functions. There are five possibilities:
- P - Programmable
- M - Multiprogrammable
- O - None
- C - Communicating
- R - Rate Modulation

The fifth letter indicates any special antitachycardial functions. There are four possibilities:
- P - Pacing (antitachyarrhythmia)
- S - Shock
- D - Dual (Pacing + Shock)
- O - None

PACEMAKER TYPES

PACEMAKER	MODE OF OPERATION	CODES
Asynchronous (also magnet mode)	Impulse discharged to atrium, ventricle, or both at preset intervals; no sensing mechanism. Used for patients without electrical activity in the atrium or ventricle. This prevents competition between the device and impulses generated by the heart, which can be fatal.	• VOO • AOO • DOO

PACEMAKER TYPES (CONTINUED)

PACEMAKER	MODE OF OPERATION	CODES
Synchronous	Stimulates ventricle by sensing activity in the atrium. If the heart rate drops below the preset optimal rate, the device discharges an impulse to the ventricle.	• VAT
Ventricular demand	Discharges at a prescribed rate when ventricle fails to discharge. Uses sensing.	• VVI • VVT
Sequential	Stimulates ventricle and atrium sequentially. Uses sensing.	• DVI • VDD
Rate-responsive	Increases rate in response activity. Senses change in ventricular stroke volume and cardiac output and adjusts rate to meet changes in demand.	• DDD • VVI, with activity
Temporary	Used in ICU for patient under constant monitoring. Can sense and fire in one chamber or both.	•VVI •DDD

*C*hapter 27. Automatic Implantable Cardioverter Defibrillator

▽   ▽   ▽   ▽   ▽   ▽   ▽

*I*NTRODUCTION

SEE TEXT PAGES

Automatic implantable cardioverter defibrillators (AICDs) correct lethal cardiac arrhythmias (ventricular fibrillation[VF] and ventricular tachycardia[VT]). The AICD is a device, surgically implanted in the abdomen, that consists of a pulse generator and sensor. Its function is to continually monitor cardiac rhythm. When an arrhythmia occurs, the device delivers a countershock.

After your patient has this device, you will need to assess how well it is working and observe your patient for adverse reactions. Therapy includes overdrive pacing, counter shock/cardioversion, and defibrillation.

*S*UPPORTING ASSESSMENT DATA

▼
▼
▼
▼
▼
▼
▼
▼
▼

▲ Health History:
Candidates for AICD therapy are persons:
• at risk for sudden cardiac death from ventricular arrhythmias (VF and VT).
• with life-threatening ventricular arrhythmias that recur and resist antiarrhythmic drug therapy.

▲ Physical Findings:
A patient having problems with an AICD may complain of the following:
• Any symptoms experienced before implantation of the device
• Any symptoms of recurrent arrhythmias

NURSE ALERT:
Make sure the patient understands that he or she should report any such symptoms immediately.

AMBULATORY CARE

When you assess an ambulatory patient who has an AICD, ask these questions:

- Do you carry medical alert indentification with your name; your physician's name, address, and phone; and your AICD settings? (Regularly remind your patient about the importance of carrying this card and wearing medical alert identification.)
- How often has the device fired?
- When did it last fire?
- How do you feel when it fires?
- What do you do after it fires?

Make sure that the patient and family can describe any adaptations they have made to the AICD. Fear and psychological maladjustment can cause ongoing problems.

Discuss activities and exercise. Remind the patient that he or she must observe certain precautions when using household items, appliances, and tools. In addition, patients must avoid the following because they may turn off the device:

- Magnets
- Stereo speakers
- Magnetic fields
- Airport security wands
- Large generators
- Power plants
- CB antennas
- Magnetic resonance imaging scans
- Maintaining or repairing electrical or gas-powered appliances

ASSESSMENT TECHNIQUES

With such patients, you should monitor the following:

- Heart rhythm
- Skin temperature
- Lung and heart sounds
- Peripheral pulses
- Antiarrhythmic drug levels
- Enzyme levels
- Electrolyte levels—especially potassium
- Patient compliance with antiarrhythmic drug therapy

TROUBLESHOOTING AICD PROBLEMS

PROBLEM	CAUSE	SOLUTION
Inappropriate firing during: • Supraventricular tachycardia • Atrial fibrillation or flutter with fast ventricular response	Heart rate beyond the VT- or VF-detect window of AICD	• Follow facility protocol to move special donut magnet over generator site to turn off the device. • Begin treatment with antiarrhythmic therapy.
Device constantly fires	• Device or lead breaks down • Electromagnetic interference • Incessant VT	• Follow institution protocol to move special donut magnet over generator site to turn off the device. • May need reprogramming
Unsuccessful defibrillation	• Energy delivery not functioning properly • Drug side effect (altered drug threshold) • Decreased ejection fraction	• Assess ABCs. • Perform CPR as needed. • May need new lead wire
VVI pacing loss of sensing	• Lead incorrectly placed • Lead dislodged • Drug side effect	• Assess ABCs. • Perform CPR as needed. • May need external pacer
VVI pacing loss of capture	• Lead incorrectly placed • Lead dislodged • Drug side effect	• Assess ABCs. • Perform CPR as needed. • May need external pacer

Chapter 28. Cardiac Catheterization, PTCA, Atherectomy, and Stents

▽   ▽   ▽   ▽   ▽   ▽   ▽

INTRODUCTION

This chapter describes various invasive procedures used to assess a patient with coronary artery disease or valvular heart disease and provides information you need to assess a patient who has recently had one of these procedures.

SUPPORTING ASSESSMENT DATA

The information that follows will help you properly assess patients who have undergone cardiac catheterization, percutaneous transluminal coronary angioplasty (PTCA), directed coronary atherectomy (DCA), or a stent insertion.

CARDIAC CATHETERIZATION
▲ Health History:

In addition to asking the appropriate questions from the Health History sections of Chapter 7, "Coronary Artery Disease," Chapter 8, "Angina Pectoris," and Chapter 9, "Myocardial Infarction," when you assess a patient who has had cardiac catheterization, ask these questions.
• When did you have your catheterization?
• Do you know the location of your blockages, if any?
• Have you ever had balloon angioplasty, bypass surgery, or any other cardiac procedure?
• Do you carry nitroglycerin?
• What medications are you currently taking?

▲ Physical Findings:

Patients with a recent catheterization may have the following symptoms:
• Hematoma
• Pain at groin site

Upon inspection and palpation, you may discover the following symptoms at the groin site. Note these symptoms because they may indicate infection.
• Drainage
• Warmth
• Tenderness

PTCA, DCA, AND STENTS
▲ Health History:
In addition to asking the appropriate questions from the Health History sections of Chapter 7, "Coronary Artery Disease," Chapter 8, "Angina Pectoris," and Chapter 9, "Myocardial Infarction," when you assess a patient who has had PTCA, DCA, or a stent, ask these questions:
- What medications are you currently taking?
- Do you carry nitroglycerin?
- Do you wear medical alert identification?
- Have you had any symptoms similar to those you had before PTCA surgery?
- Have you ever participated in a cardiac rehabilitation program?
- Do you smoke?
- When did you last have an exercise stress test?

▲ Physical Findings:
Patients with a recent history of these procedures may have the following symptoms:
- Chest pain that does not respond to nitroglycerin
- Decreased exercise tolerance
- An increase in shortness of breath
- Fainting

NURSE ALERT:
Make sure the patient understands that any of these symptoms are potentially serious and should be reported immediately. They may reflect reocclusion of the artery.

The most serious complication is abrupt reclosure of the coronary artery after PTCA. This occurs in approximately 4% of patients within a few hours of the procedure. It can be life-threatening. Such patients may have the following symptoms:
- Symptoms of myocardial infarction (see Chapter 9, "Myocardial Infarction"), including tachycardia, chest pain, anxiety, and diaphoresis
- An ECG that shows changes in ST and T waves, such as those seen in myocardial ischemia (see Chapter 9, "Myocardial Infarction")

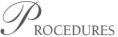PROCEDURES

All of these procedures are invasive. Some are used to assess the extent of the patient's disease, others to correct problems caused by the disease.

Cardiac Catheterization

Cardiac catheterization is used to assess the patient. A radiopaque catheter, inserted through a peripheral vessel, usually in the femoral artery in the groin, is threaded into the heart. When assessing the left ventricle, this procedure measures pressure and cardiac output to support a diagnosis of valvular stenosis or resistance. Fluoroscopy with dye provides visualization of the heart chambers, valves, and coronary arteries. This procedure measures pulmonary vascular pressure. It can be used to perform the following:

- Identify the location and severity of coronary artery lesions
- Assess valvular disease, atrial septal defects
- Measure heart pressures and assess left ventricular function
- Measure cardiac output and ejection fraction
- Measure blood gases

PTCA

Percutaneous transluminal coronary angioplasty can be a nonsurgical alternative to bypass surgery for some patients.The narrowed coronary lumen is dilated with a balloon catheter. The inflated balloon compresses plaque into the vessel wall. PTCA is appropriate for patients with the following history:

- Documented myocardial ischemia
- Proximal lesion of one artery
- Multivessel disease in select cases
- Acute myocardial infarction
- Completely occluded artery, in some cases
- Previous bypass surgery
- At high risk for complications with bypass

There is always the possibility that bypass surgery will be required.

The best candidate for PTCA is a patient who has had severe angina for less than 1 year. He or she is likely to have noncalcified, concentric, discrete, smooth lesions. These lesions are soft and much easier to work with.

Patients at risk for abrupt reclosure include those with complicated lesions and those involving a thrombus that occurs at an acute angle or at a branching point of the coronary artery. This risk of reocclusion is the greatest in the first 6 months following the procedure. About 30% to 50% of PTCA patients need a second intervention.

Additional complications can include myocardial infarction, arterial spasm, hemorrhaging, insufficient circulation, hypokalemia, arrhythmias, hypotension, restenosis within 2 to 6 months, and renal intolerance to contrast material.

Atherectomy

Directed coronary atherectomy is a procedure in some ways similar to PTCA. The catheter has a tiny cutting blade, a collection chamber, and a balloon. Plaque is cut away from the lumen of the artery, clearing a smoother surface than with a PTCA. Selection of this modality depends on the location and character of the vessel and the plaque.

Stents

Stents are small, metal mesh tubes used to keep a coronary artery open after PTCA. The insertion of the stent can help some patients have improved patency, thus reducing the need for a bypass. Because the stent is a foreign substance, medication to decrease the incidence of clotting is used for the first few months after the stent procedure. Stents reduce the incidence of restenosis after angioplasty by as much as 35%.

$\mathscr{C}$hapter 29. Coronary Artery Bypass Grafting

▽   ▽   ▽   ▽   ▽   ▽   ▽

$\mathscr{I}$NTRODUCTION

SEE TEXT PAGES

Coronary artery bypass grafting (CABG), is a surgical procedure that bypasses a blocked coronary artery using a segment of a vein (usually the saphenous vein from the leg) or an artery (left or right, internal or mammary). Remember: Patients with a history of CABG have coronary artery disease, which is progressive. The longer it has been since the surgery, the more likely it is that grafts may occlude. Take a careful history of symptoms. Pay particular attention to symptoms listed in Chapter 8, "Angina Pectoris," and Chapter 9, "Myocardial Infarction."

$\mathscr{S}$UPPORTING ASSESSMENT DATA

The information that follows will help you properly assess patients who have undergone CABG.

▲ Health History:

Patients who have severe angina (see Chapter 8, "Angina Pectoris") or a myocardial infarction (see Chapter 9, "Myocardial Infarction") are most likely to undergo CABG. Other candidates include patients whose heart disease substantially affects their quality of life. CABG can alleviate symptoms and eliminate or decrease myocardial ischemia.

▲ Physical Findings:

The most likely complication of CABG is stenosis of the grafts. The following symptoms may suggest occluded graft vessels or new disease:
- Symptoms of angina pectoris as described in Chapter 8, "Angina Pectoris"
- Symptoms the patient experienced prior to surgery
- Symptoms of MI as described in Chapter 9, "Myocardial Infarction"

NURSE ALERT:
Remind your postoperative patient to call immediately if he or she experiences one or more of the following:
- Fever
- Muscle pain
- Sore throat
- Redness, edema, or drainage from any incision
- Joint pain
- Dizziness
- Angina
- Abnormal pulse
- Reduced exercise tolerance
- Weakness

AMBULATORY CARE

When you assess an ambulatory CABG patient, ask these questions:
- When did you have your surgery?
- How many grafts do you have?
- What medication do you take?
- Do you carry nitroglycerin?
- Do you wear medical alert identification?
- Have you had any post operative symptoms similar to those you had before the surgery?
- Have you ever attended a cardiac rehabilitation program?
- Do you exercise regularly?
- Do you follow a low-fat diet?
- Do you smoke?
- When was your last exercise stress test?

THE PROCEDURE

Coronary artery bypass grafting has become a common procedure. Its function is to save a patient with acute or chronic ischemia caused by myocardial infarction. CABG involves taking a segment of saphenous vein from the leg or the mammary artery and using it to bypass the damaged and blocked artery. This restores normal blood flow to the heart. The preferred method involves rerouting a mammary artery. This saves the patient an incision in the leg and has a better patency record.

In either case, the surgeon attaches one end of the graft to the aorta and the other end to the damaged artery just below the blockage. An alternative method with a mammary or gastroepiploic artery is to leave one end of the graft attached to the originating artery and sew the other just below the blockage on the damaged artery. Coronary blood flow travels through the graft, bypassing the blockage. This restores normal blood flow and oxygen delivery to the heart.

Chapter 30. Orthotopic Heart Transplantation

▽ ▽ ▽ ▽ ▽ ▽ ▽

INTRODUCTION

SEE TEXT PAGES

In an orthotopic heart transplantation, the surgical team removes the recipient's heart and replaces it with one from a donor.

SUPPORTING ASSESSMENT DATA

The information that follows will help you properly assess patients who have undergone orthotopic heart transplantation.

▲ Health History:

A patient who suffers from severe coronary artery disease or other degenerative heart disease who has no other viable treatment alternative is a candidate for orthotopic heart transplantation. Without the transplant, such an individual would not live more than 6 months to 1 year.

▲ Physical Findings:

When you assess a patient who has had a heart transplant, your primary concern will be to check for symptoms of rejection. The risk of rejection peaks during the first 18 days after surgery. Remember: Immunosuppressant drugs mask the symptoms of acute rejection until it is quite advanced.

- Acute rejection appears in the first 3 months after surgery. The majority of transplant patients experience at least two episodes of acute rejection, which is diagnosed with an endomyocardial biopsy.
- Chronic rejection can occur any time after 3 months. Its symptoms are the same as those for coronary artery disease (see Chapter 7, "Coronary Artery Disease"). It results in ischemic myocardial damage. Patients must have regular endomyocardial biopsies, exercise stress tests, and cardiac catheterization to rule out chronic rejection.

NURSE ALERT:
Because the donor heart is cut off from direct sympathetic stimulation, you will not see classic angina symptoms.

On the patient's ECG, expect to see two P waves (one is a remnant) because the patient has two sinoatrial nodes (one from the original heart and one from the recipient heart).

*A*MBULATORY CARE

When assessing an ambulatory recipient of orthotopic heart transplantation, ask these questions:
• How long have you had your new heart?
• Which transplant center follows your progress?
• When was your last myocardial biopsy and what were the results?
• Do you wear medical alert identification?
• Have you had any episodes of rejection?
• What medications do you currently take?
• Have you ever attended a cardiac rehabilitation program?
• Do you exercise regularly and follow a low-fat diet?

*T*RANSPLANTATION TECHNIQUES

There are two types of transplantation techniques—orthotopic and heterotopic.
• In orthotopic transplantation, the donor heart replaces the recipient heart. The recipient's atrial septum as well as the posterior and lateral walls of the atria remain in place and serve to "anchor" the new heart. The surgeon clips the atria on the donor heart so that the anterior atrial walls, sinoatrial node, and internodal conduction pathways are kept intact. The surgeon then connects the recipient and donor atria, pulmonary arteries, and aortas.
• In heterotopic transplantation, the donor heart "piggy-backs"on the recipient heart. The donor heart is placed next to the recipient heart and they are connected between the left and right atria, aortas, and pulmonary arteries with a synthetic graft. This procedure is only used for patients with such severe pulmonary hypertension that the donor heart could not pump alone. In rare instances, it is also used when the patient is terminal and the donor heart is too small.

Whichever transplantation technique is used, the patient must receive immunosuppressant drug therapy for the rest of his or her life. This therapy is usually a combination of prednisone, cyclosporine, and azathioprine. This allows the patient's physician to adjust each drug to reduce side effects. These patients must be monitored by their transplant center for life.

Suggested Readings

Arato, A., et al. "Elderly Care: Automatic Implantable Cardioverter Defibrillators." *Journal of Gerontological Nursing* 18 (December 1992): 15–34.

Arteaga, W. J., and B. J. Drew. "Device Therapy for Ventricular Tachycardia or Fibrillation: The Implantable Cardioverter Defibrillator and Antitachycardiac Pacing." *Critical Care Quarterly* 14 (1991): 60–71.

Brown, A. "Discharge Functional Capacity and Self-Efficacy of Men After Coronary Artery Bypass Graft Surgery." *Canadian Journal of Cardiovascular Medicine* 3 (September-December 1992): 18–24.

Mercer, M. E. "Electrical Support for the Heart: Rate-Responsive Pacers." *RN* 55 (May 1992): 34–37.

Stafford, M. J., and K. M. Kleinschmidt. "Physiological Cardiac Pacing: The DDD Pacemaker System and Rate-Responsive Modes." *Cardiovascular Nursing* 27 (1991): 13–18.

SECTION VIII. CARDIAC COMPLICATIONS

Chapter 31. Cardiogenic and Noncardiogenic Shock

▽   ▽   ▽   ▽   ▽   ▽   ▽

INTRODUCTION

SEE TEXT PAGES

Cardiogenic shock occurs secondary to some other cardiac condition. The prognosis for patients with cardiogenic shock is poor. Noncardiogenic shock occurs secondary to an allergic reaction, an infection, or hypovolemia. All types of shock reduce tissue perfusion and cellular anoxia occurs.

SUPPORTING ASSESSMENT DATA

If your assessment findings are similar to those listed here, they may suggest cardiogenic or noncardiogenic shock.

▲ Health History:

Consider at risk for cardiogenic shock patients who have any condition that reduces left ventricular function, such as myocardial infarction, cardiac tamponade, or myocardial injury.

Consider at risk for hypovolemic shock patients who have:
• Lost 20% or more blood volume due to external or internal injury or an internal disease process, like pancreatitis
• Dehydration
• Diabetes insipidus
• A GI problem, such as an obstruction or peritonitis
• Recent diuresis
• Cirrhosis of the liver
• Pancreatitis

Consider at risk for septic shock patients who have:
• Had or have an infection, most commonly *Escherichia coli, Klebsiella pneumoniae, Serratia, Enterobacteria,* or *Pseudomonas*
• Burn injuries
• Wounds or catheters
• Septicemia
• Chronic coronary disease

- Malnutrition
- Excessive stress
- A history of alcoholism
- Bone marrow suppression
- Used or use antibiotics excessively
- Or have had a fungal infection

Consider at risk for anaphylactic shock patients who have a severe allergic reaction.

▲ Physical Findings:

Patients in the early stages of shock will have the following symptoms, regardless of the cause:

- Nausea
- Weakness
- Thirst
- Restlessness
- Hypotension

Patients in the later stages of shock will have the following symptoms, regardless of the cause:

- Hypothermia
- Drowsiness
- Respiratory distress
- Diaphoresis
- Confusion
- Fatigue and lethargy
- Diminished or absent urine output

SHOCK SYMPTOMS AND COMPLAINTS

CARDIOGENIC	HYPOVOLEMIC	SEPTIC	ANAPHYLACTIC
• Angina	• Angina-like pain • Acute tubular necrosis • Renal failure • Multisystem organ failure • Intravascular coagulation	• Fever • Chills • Bounding pulse	• Difficulty breathing • Urticaria • Nausea and vomiting • Diarrhea • Dizziness

!

NURSE ALERT:
20% of patients in hyperdynamic septic shock are likely to have symptoms of hypothermia.

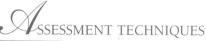 SSESSMENT TECHNIQUES

 Use inspection, palpation, and auscultation to assess the patient. The following table describes common results you may find with any type of shock using these techniques. Note: Orthostatic vital signs and tilt test may be useful for detecting shock.

COMMON ASSESSMENT FINDINGS

INSPECTION	AUSCULTATION	PALPATION
• Pale, cool, clammy, skin • Cyanosis • Decreased sensorium • Rapid, shallow respirations • Substantially reduced or absent urine output • Dry, pale mucous membrane • Restlessness, irritability, anxiety, short attention span (early stages) • Apathy, confusion, lethargy, coma (late stages) • Hyperventilation • Hypothermia	• Mean arterial pressure less than 60 mm Hg • Narrowing pulse pressure	• Rapid, irregular, thready peripheral pulses

SHOCK SYMPTOMS

INSPECTION	
Cardiogenic	• Distended neck veins • Peripheral edema
Hypovolemic	• Flat neck veins • Cardiac output <4 to 8 liters/min.
Septic	• Hyperdynamic - pink skin - warm skin - flushing

SHOCK SYMPTOMS *(CONTINUED)*

INSPECTION

Septic *(continued)*	• Hypodynamic
	  - pale, cool skin
	  - cyanotic mottling of skin
	  - coma

Anaphylactic	• Urticaria • Seizures • Angioedema

AUSCULTATION

Cardiogenic	• Drop in blood pressure • Galloping heartbeat • Faint heart sounds • Crackles • Dyspnea • Rarely, a holosystolic murmur
Hypovolemic	• Right atrial pressure <1 to 6 mm Hg • Pulmonary artery pressure <10 to 20 mm Hg • Pulmonary artery wedge pressure <6 to 12 mm Hg

Septic	• Hyperdynamic (normal or slightly elevated blood pressure)
	• Hypodynamic
	  - hypotension
	  - lung crackles

Anaphylactic	• Drop in pressure • Arrhythmias • Wheezing

SHOCK SYMPTOMS *(CONTINUED)*

PALPATION	
Cardiogenic	• Increased heart rate
Hypovolemic	• Rapid, thready peripheral pulses • Cold, clammy skin
Septic	• Hyperdynamic (rapid full peripheral pulses; weak, rapid, or absent peripheral pulse; warm, dry skin)
Anaphylactic	• Increase in heart rate • Reduced or absent peripheral pulses

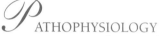

𝒫ATHOPHYSIOLOGY

Each type of shock has a different mechanism.
- The mechanisms for cardiogenic shock are any conditions that cause cardiac failure, such as a myocardial infarction or myocardial injury.
- The mechanisms for hypovolemic shock include conditions that reduce intravascular blood volume by at least 20%. Blood volume can no longer meet the demands of tissue metabolism.
- The mechanisms for anaphylactic shock are anything that causes an allergic reaction, such as a bee sting, blood transfusion, or medication.
- The mechanisms for septic shock are any bacterial, viral, or fungal pathogens that cause a systemic infection.

No matter the type of shock, it is a potentially life-threatening condition. The body responds to shock with compensatory mechanisms in an effort to maintain cardiac output and organ tissue perfusion and function. The outcome is decreased cellular profusion followed by cellular hypoxia and, finally, organ failure and death.

It is imperative to detect shock quickly. Early intervention markedly increases the patient's chances for survival. After shock occurs, the pathophysiology is the same.

THE PROGRESSION OF SHOCK

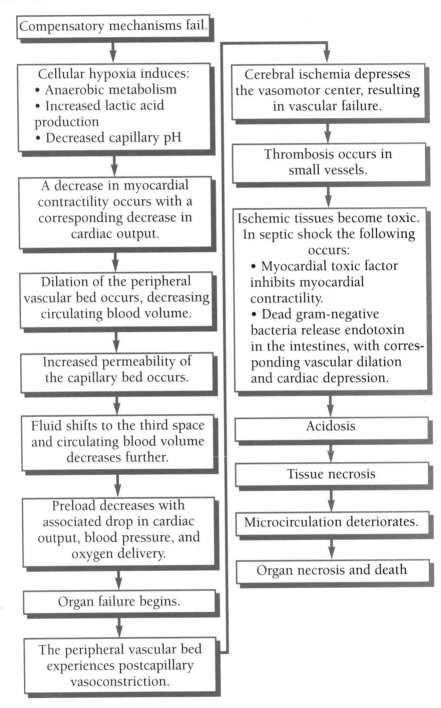

Compensatory mechanisms fail.

Cellular hypoxia induces:
• Anaerobic metabolism
• Increased lactic acid production
• Decreased capillary pH

A decrease in myocardial contractility occurs with a corresponding decrease in cardiac output.

Dilation of the peripheral vascular bed occurs, decreasing circulating blood volume.

Increased permeability of the capillary bed occurs.

Fluid shifts to the third space and circulating blood volume decreases further.

Preload decreases with associated drop in cardiac output, blood pressure, and oxygen delivery.

Organ failure begins.

The peripheral vascular bed experiences postcapillary vasoconstriction.

Cerebral ischemia depresses the vasomotor center, resulting in vascular failure.

Thrombosis occurs in small vessels.

Ischemic tissues become toxic. In septic shock the following occurs:
• Myocardial toxic factor inhibits myocardial contractility.
• Dead gram-negative bacteria release endotoxin in the intestines, with corresponding vascular dilation and cardiac depression.

Acidosis

Tissue necrosis

Microcirculation deteriorates.

Organ necrosis and death

𝒞hapter 32. Cardiac Arrhythmias and Conduction Disturbances

▽ ▽ ▽ ▽ ▽ ▽ ▽

𝒥NTRODUCTION

Cardiac arrhythmias are conduction disturbances that disrupt the normal functioning of the heart. The symptoms associated with arrhythmias are related to decreased cardiac output. Heart rates above 150/min (supraventricular tachycardia, ventricular tachycardia) or below 50/min (bradycardia, second and third degree heart block, and frequent premature ventricular contractions) often result in hypoperfusion due to reduced cardiac output.

Your assessment should focus on detecting signs of hypofusion (the result of decreased cardiac output), such as dizziness, light-headedness, change in level of consciousness to unconsciousness or syncope (hypoxia to the brain), or chest pressure, pain (angina), dyspnea, and a drop in blood pressure due to reduced cardiac output and systemic circulation.

Generalized symptoms of reduced cardiac output can be fatigue, inability to do work (such as walking up steps), and just not feeling well.

NURSE ALERT:

Do not be quick to treat the patient with an arrhythmia who is asymptomatic. Instead, focus on assessing for underlying causes, such as ischemia and medication effects (as in drug toxicity). The goal is to prevent the arrhythmia from progressing, causing a fall in cardiac output that will cause symptoms.

𝒮UPPORTING ASSESSMENT DATA

If your assessment findings are similar to those listed here, they may suggest cardiac arrhythmias or conduction disturbances.

▲ Health History:

Arrhythmias and conduction defects can be precipitated by coronary artery disease (CAD), myocardial infarction (MI), hypertensive disease, and drug therapy with digitalis or quinidine.

▲ Physical Findings:

Signs and symptoms of cardiac arrhythmias are idiosyncratic. Other than light-headedness and syncope, many patients with arrhythmia defects are asymptomatic, whereas others are in cardiac arrest. Common symptoms are as follows:

- Alteration in level of consciousness
- Vertigo
- Dizziness and fainting
- Seizures
- Weakness and fatigue
- Exercise intolerance
- Dyspnea
- Chest pain
- Palpitations
- Feeling of "skipped beats"
- Anxiety
- Restlessness

COMMON SYMPTOMS

INSPECTION	AUSCULTATION	PALPATION
• Dusky or pale skin	• Crackles • Abnormal heart rate • Abnormal blood pressure • Abnormal heart sounds • Abnormal respiratory rate	• Paradoxical pulses • Irregular pulse • Palpable skipped beats • Cool, clammy skin

PRECIPITATING FACTORS

ARRHYTHMIA	ETIOLOGY
Sinus arrhythmia	• Normal in athletes, children, and elderly patients • Altered vagal tone; MI • Digitalis toxicity

PRECIPITATING FACTORS (CONTINUED)

ARRHYTHMIA	ETIOLOGY
Sinus tachycardia	• Fever, exercise, anxiety, pain, fluid loss, shock • Left ventricular failure, cardiac tamponade, anterior wall MI • Pulmonary embolism • Hyperthyroidism • Anemia • Hypovolemia • Any atropine-like drug, caffeine, alcohol, nicotine, epinephrine
Sinus bradycardia	• Normal in athletes • Increased intracranial pressure, bowel straining, vomiting, intubation, mechanical ventilation • Sick sinus syndrome • Hypothyroidism • Inferior wall MI, Valsalva's maneuver (increased vagal tone) • Medications such as beta blockers, digitalis glycosides, morphine
Sinoatrial arrest or block	• Infection • CAD, inferior wall MI, vagal stimulation, Valsalva's maneuver, carotid sinus massage • Medications such as digitalis (toxicity) and quinidine • Salicylate toxicity • Pesticide poisoning • Endotracheal intubation • Sick sinus syndrome
Wandering atrial pacemaker	• Rheumatic carditis • Digitalis toxicity • Sick sinus syndrome

PRECIPITATING FACTORS *(CONTINUED)*

ARRHYTHMIA	ETIOLOGY
Premature atrial contraction	• CAD, atrial ischemia, heart failure, atherosclerosis • Acute respiratory failure, chronic obstructive pulmonary disease (COPD) • Electrolyte imbalance • Hypoxia • Digitalis toxicity • Medications like aminophylline and adrenergics • Caffeine, nicotine • Anxiety, stress, fatigue
Paroxysmal atrial tachycardia	• Abnormality of atrioventricular (AV) conduction system • Stress • Hypoxia • Hypokalemia • Cardiomyopathy, congenital heart disease, MI, valvular disease, Wolff-Parkinson-White syndrome, cor pulmonale • Hyperthyroidism • Systemic hypertension • Digitalis toxicity • Caffeine, marijuana, nicotine, other CNS stimulants
Atrial flutter	• Heart failure, CAD, tricuspid valve disease, mitral valve disease, cardiac surgery, inferior wall MI, myocarditis • Pulmonary embolism, cor pulmonale

PRECIPITATING FACTORS *(CONTINUED)*

ARRHYTHMIA	ETIOLOGY
Atrial fibrillation	• Heart failure, COPD, constrictive pericarditis, ischemic heart disease, congestive heart failure, mitral stenosis, atrial irritation, coronary bypass or valve replacement complication • Hypertension • Sepsis • Digitalis toxicity (rare) • Thyrotoxicosis • Hypertension • Digitalis glycoside, nifedipine
Junctional rhythm	• Inferior wall MI, inferior wall ischemia, vagal stimulation, valve surgery, sick sinus syndrome • Rheumatic fever • Hyperkalemia • Digitalis toxicity
Premature junctional contractions	• MI • Ischemia • Digitalis toxicity • Caffeine and amphetamines
First-degree AV block	• Can be normal in healthy patient • Inferior wall MI, ischemia, CAD, increased vagal tone, congenital anomalies • Hypothyroidism • Hypokalemia • Hyperkalemia • Digitalis toxicity • Medication such as quinidine, procainamide, propranolol

PRECIPITATING FACTORS *(CONTINUED)*

ARRHYTHMIA	ETIOLOGY
Second-degree AV block; Mobitz I	• Inferior wall MI, cardiac surgery, vagal stimulation • Rheumatic fever • Digitalis toxicity • Quinidine, procainamide, propranolol
Second-degree AV block; Mobitz II	• Anterior wall MI, ischemia, CAD, myocarditis • Digitalis toxicity
Third-degree AV block; complete heart block	• Inferior or anterior wall MI, congenital abnormality, conduction system fibrosis or degeneration, myocarditis, cardiac surgery • Rheumatic fever • Hypoxia • Connective tissue fibrosis • Digitalis toxicity
Junctional tachycardia	• Inferior wall MI, myocarditis, cardiomyopathy, inferior wall ischemia, valve replacement • Rheumatic fever • Digitalis toxicity
Premature ventricular contractions (PVCs)	• Heart failure, myocardial ischemia, MI, CAD, myocardial contusion, ventricular catheter complication • Hypoxia • Hypokalemia • Hypocalcemia • Acidosis • Drug toxicity • Caffeine, tobacco, alcohol • Stress (anxiety or pain) • Exercise

PRECIPITATING FACTORS (*CONTINUED*)

ARRHYTHMIA	ETIOLOGY
Ventricular tachycardia	• Myocardial ischemia, MI, ventricular aneurysm, CAD, rheumatic heart disease, mitral valve prolapse, heart failure, cardiomyopathy, ventricular catheter, pulmonary embolism • Hypokalemia • Hypercalcemia • Hypoxia • Drug toxicity • Anxiety
Torsades de Pointes	• Drug toxicity • Hypokalemia • Hypomagnesemia
Ventricular fibrillation	• Myocardial ischemia, MI (most often), ventricular tachycardia, R-on-T phenomenon • Electric shock • Hypothermia • Hyperkalemia • Hypercalcemia
Ventricular standstill	• Alkalosis • Myocardial ischemia, MI, aortic valve disease, heart failure, ventricular aneurysms, atrioventricular arrhythmias, AV block, heart rupture, cardiac tamponade, electromechanical dissociation • Electric shock • Hypoxemia • Hypokalemia • Hyperkalemia • Cocaine overdose
Bundle branch block	• Myocardial fibrosis, CAD, MI, congenital anomalies • Pulmonary embolism

DIAGNOSTIC TESTS

TEST	FINDINGS
Drug levels	Toxic agent (digitalis, cocaine, and so on)
12-Lead ECG	• Arrhythmias • Essential bundle branch blocks
Serum electrolytes	• Hypokalemia • Hypomagnesemia • Hypocalcemia • Hyperkalemia **NURSE ALERT:** Do not treat arrhythmias with lidocaine in the presence of decreased potassium, magnesium, or calcium levels.
24-hr. Holter monitoring	Arrhythmia summary and frequency
Cardiac event recorder	Arrhythmia related to patient's symptoms
Cardiac catheterization	Underlying ischemia
Electrophysiologic studies	Inducibility
Exercise stress test (with 24-hr. Holter monitoring)	• Target heart rate • Stress point at which symptoms appear

ECG CRITERIA AND FINDINGS

The following table lists criteria specific to each type of arrhythmia. You will generally use a single-lead or multi-lead ECG strip. Bundle branch blocks require a 12-lead ECG.

ARRHYTHMIA	FINDINGS
Sinus arrhythmia 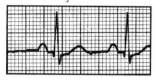	• Irregular atrial and ventricular rhythms • Normal P wave before each QRS complex • Normal heart rate 60–100 beats/min
Sinus tachycardia 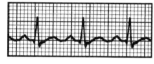	• Regular atrial rhythm • Rate 100 to 150 beats/min • Normal PQRST
Sinus bradycardia 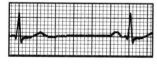	• Regular atrial and ventricular rates • Rate <60 beats/min • Normal PQRST
Sinoatrial arrest 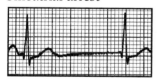	• Normal QRST • Varying R-R intervals (arrest) • Pause after preceding beat (arrest) • Heart rate normal or <60 beats/min • P wave missing for arrested beat • Beat after pause is on time
Sinoatrial block 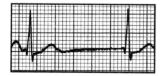	• Normal atrial and ventricular rhythm, with exception of missing complex (block) • Heart rate normal or <60 beats/min • No PQRST for blocked beat • Interval before and after pause is twice normal • May see junctional or ventricular escape beats

ECG CRITERIA AND FINDINGS (*CONTINUED*)

ARRHYTHMIA	FINDINGS

Sick sinus syndrome
(or tachycardia-bradycardia
syndrome)

NURSE ALERT:
You may frequently see sick sinus syndrome, which is a combination of sinus arrhythmias. The cardiac output falls, often causing syncope. The Sinoatrial node fails and escape pacemakers no longer initiate impulses.

Wandering atrial pacemaker

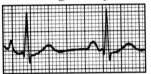

• Minor variations in atrial and ventricular rates
• PR interval irregular, but not prolonged
• P waves irregular (different morphology)
• QRS beat irregular (follows the atrial complex)

Premature atrial contraction

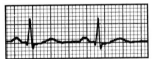

• Irregular rhythm, ectopic beat disrupts underlying rhythm
• Abnormal, early P waves
• P waves followed by QRS complexes
• QRS complex may be normal, abnormal, or absent after the PAC
• P wave can appear in preceding T wave or be buried in it

Paroxysmal atrial tachycardia

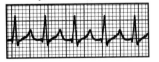

• Regular atrial and ventricular rates
• Irregular rhythm
• Heart rate between 150 and 250 beats/min
• Regular P waves but may be hard to distinguish from T waves
• R-R interval abnormal
• Starts and stops abruptly

ECG CRITERIA AND FINDINGS *(CONTINUED)*

ARRHYTHMIA	FINDINGS
Supraventricular tachycardia 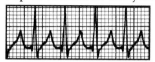	• Heart rate >150 beats/min • Regular rhythm • P waves can't be seen • Has no left-axis deviation • QRS complex peaks symmetrically • No rS configuration in V_6 • If underlying QRS is wide due to Bundle branch block, ventricular tachycardia is hard to differentiate • Need 12-lead ECG—Look at V_1 and V_6 **NURSE ALERT:** Assess symptoms using advanced cardiac life support (ACLS) protocols.
Multifocal atrial tachycardia 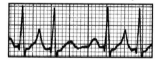	• Atrial rhythm irregular • Heart rate 100 to 150 beats/min • Wide variance in P-P and R-R intervals • Wide variance in P-wave morphology
Atrial flutter 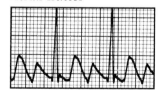	• Regular atrial rhythm • Variable ventricular rhythm • Atrial rate (F waves), if able to count, is 250 to 350 beats/min • Sawtooth P waves • Uniformly shaped QRS complexes but rate is irregular
Atrial fibrillation 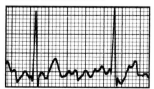	• Irregular atrial rhythm; atrial rate >400 beats/min, no pattern • Ventricular rate 60-100 if controlled; <60 or >100 if uncontrolled • Extremely irregular ventricular rate • Uniform QRS complexes • No apparent PR interval • No P waves (if present, erratic)

ECG CRITERIA AND FINDINGS *(CONTINUED)*

ARRHYTHMIA	FINDINGS
Junctional rhythm 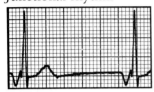	• Regular atrial and ventricular rates • Ectopic beat disrupts underlying rhythm • Ventricular rate 40 to 60 beats/min • P waves may be absent, precede, hide in, or follow QRS complex • Atrial rate 40 to 60 beats/min • P waves often inverted • PR interval <0.12 second or absent • QRS complex normal, with exception of aberrant conduction
Premature junctional contractions 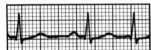	• Irregular atrial and ventricular rhythms, depend on frequency • Ectopic beat disrupts underlying rhythm • PR interval precedes, hides in, or follows QRS complex, often inverted. • When P wave precedes QRS complex, interval <0.12 second • Normal QRS complex
First-degree AV block 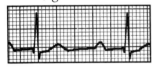	• Regular atrial and ventricular rhythms • Rate 60 to 100 beats/min • PR interval >0.20 second • P wave before each QRS complex • QRS complex normal
Second-degree AV block; Mobitz I (Wenckebach) 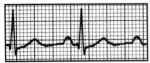	• Normal atrial rhythm • Rate usually <60 beats/min • Grouped beating cycle • Progressively longer PR intervals until a QRS complex is missing • R-R shortens as PR lengthens • P-P interval constant and regular • Irregular ventricular rhythm • Atrial rate greater than ventricular rate • PR interval shortens after dropped beat • Normal QRS complex

ECG CRITERIA AND FINDINGS (CONTINUED)

ARRHYTHMIA	FINDINGS
Second-degree AV block; Mobitz II 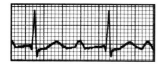	• Regular atrial rhythm • P-P interval constant • P wave pause twice RR interval • PR interval constant (usually >0.20 second) for conducted beats • Atrial to ventricular response 2:1 or 3:1 conduction • Irregular or regular ventricular rate • QRS complexes periodically absent
Third-degree AV block 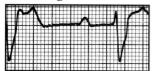	• Regular atrial rate 60 to 100 beats/min • Regular P-P intervals • Regular R-R interval • Slow and regular ventricular rate 40 to 60 beats/min if escape focus is junctional, 20-60 if ventricular • No relation between P waves and QRS complexes • No constant PR interval • QRS interval normal or wide and abnormal; <0.12 second if junctional, >0.12 second if ventricular
Junctional tachycardia 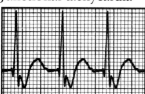	• Atrial rate <100 beats/min, but P waves often absent, hidden in QRS complex, or before T wave • Ventricular rate 100 to 160 beats/min • Inverted P wave • Normal QRS configuration <0.12 sec • Sudden onset of rhythm, often in bursts
Premature ventricular contractions 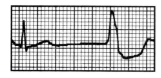	• Regular atrial rate • Ectopic beat disrupts underlying rhythm • Irregular ventricular rate • Premature QRS complex, followed by compensatory pause • QRS complex wide and abnormal, generally >0.14 second for ectopic beat • Premature QRS complexes, singly, paired, or in threes • Unifocal—all PVCs look the same • Multifocal—different morphologies

ECG CRITERIA AND FINDINGS (CONTINUED)

ARRHYTHMIA	FINDINGS

Premature ventricular
contractions (continued)

NURSE ALERT:
Frequent, multifocal PVCs, couplets, triplets, or R-on-T wave PVCs can predispose a patient to ventricular fibrillation and ventricular tachycardia. Assess symptoms and underlying causes. May need treatment.

Ventricular tachycardia

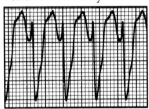

- Ventricular rate 140 to 220 beats/min
- Extremely abnormal and wide QRS complexes with no relation to P waves
- Regular or irregular ventricular rate
- Left-axis deviation >30 degrees
- Three or more consecutive PVCs
- QRS complex left peak taller than right for lead V_1
- Episode begins with PVC
- V_6 shows rS configuration
- P waves absent, or visible in QRS complex
- May start and stop with no apparent pattern

NURSE ALERT:
If pulseless, assess ABCs of CPR. Assess symptoms and follow ACLS protocols.

ECG CRITERIA AND FINDINGS (CONTINUED)

ARRHYTHMIA	FINDINGS
Torsades de Pointes 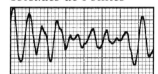	• Irregular, wide QRS complex changed by twisting along isoelectric axis • QT interval > 0.50 second • Prominent U waves • Heart rate 150 to 250 beats/min **NURSE ALERT:** Do not treat with lidocaine; it will worsen arrhythmia.
Ventricular fibrillation 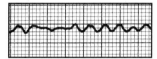	• Rapid, chaotic ventricular rhythm • Abnormal, wide QRS complexes • Fine or coarse • P waves absent **NURSE ALERT:** If pulseless, assess ABCs of CPR. Assess symptoms and follow ACLS protocols.
Ventricular asystole 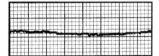	• Flat ECG with no QRS complex **NURSE ALERT:** If pulseless, assess ABCs of CPR. Assess symptoms and follow ACLS protocols.
Left bundle branch block 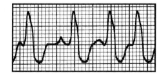	• Wide QRS complex • V_1 shows negative QRS complex or rS pattern • V_6 positive QRS with broad R wave • Q wave and S wave absent in leads I, aVL, V_5, V_6. Note: Must have a 12-lead ECG.

ECG CRITERIA AND FINDINGS (CONTINUED)

ARRHYTHMIA	FINDINGS
Right bundle branch block 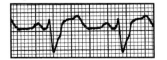	• QRS complex >0.12 second • Leads I, aVL, V₄ show broad S waves • Triphasic QRS complex with rSR1 configuration in lead V1 • Triphasic QRS complex with qRS configuration in lead V₆ Note: Must have a 12-lead ECG.
Left anterior hemiblock 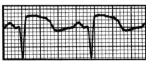	• Leads II, III, and aVF show small R and S waves • Leads I and aVL show small Q and R waves • QRS at upper-duration limits Note: Must have a 12-lead ECG.
Left posterior hemiblock 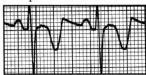	• Leads II, III, and aVF show small Q and tall R waves • Leads I and VR show small R and tall S waves • Right axis deviation ≥120 degrees Note: Must have a 12-lead ECG.

$\mathcal{O}$THER DIAGNOSTIC TOOLS

The following blood studies are also useful as diagnostic tools:
• Creatine kinase
• Lactate dehydrogenase
• Aspartate aminotransferase
• Hydroxybutyric dehydrogenase
• Lipoprotein fractionation
• Serum electrolytes
• Blood gas analysis

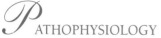

PATHOPHYSIOLOGY

Arrhythmias usually result from CAD, ischemia, MI, and other conditions that interfere with electrical initiation and/or conduction. They can be so mild that they require no care or so severe that they are life-threatening. They are classified by origin in the heart—atrial, junctional, or ventricular. The source of the arrhythmia affects cardiac output and blood pressure. Even when your patient's heart is healthy, the rapid and irregular rhythms of an arrhythmia can cause strain or damage.

There are different mechanisms that cause arrhythmias.
- Disturbance in automaticity: Your patient has a disturbance in automaticity when the sinus node or another site in the atria, AV junction, or ventricles has enhanced ability to initiate an impulse. Ischemia and drug effects can increase or decrease automaticity. This may cause premature beats and abnormal rhythms.
- Disturbances in conductivity: When the passage of the electrical impulse occurs too rapidly (as with supraventricular tachycardia, or re-entry tachycardia) or is slowed or blocked (as with AV block), your patient has a disturbance in conductivity.

Chapter 33. Cardiac Tamponade

▽   ▽   ▽   ▽   ▽   ▽   ▽

INTRODUCTION

SEE TEXT PAGES

Cardiac tamponade occurs whenever the pressure in the pericardial sac rises too quickly, impairing diastolic filling.

SUPPORTING ASSESSMENT DATA

If your assessment findings are similar to those listed here, they may suggest cardiac tamponade.

▲ Health History:

In addition to the health risk factors listed in Chapter 7, "Coronary Artery Disease," consider at risk patients who have a history of the following:

- Dressler's syndrome
- Cancer (pericardial effusion)
- Bacterial infection
- Tuberculosis
- Hemorrhage from a wound or injury
- Recent cardiac catheterization or surgery
- Pericarditis
- Myocardial infarction
- Chronic renal failure
- Drug reaction
- Connective tissue disease
- Rheumatic fever (rare)

▲ Physical Findings:

Patients with cardiac tamponade are likely to have the following symptoms:

- Acute pain that eases when leaning forward in a sitting position
- Dyspnea

AMBULATORY CARE

When assessing the ambulatory patient, ask the patient if he or she has ever had pericardiocentesis and why.

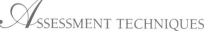SSESSMENT TECHNIQUES

On inspection, the patient may appear:
- Diaphoretic
- Orthopneic
- Anxious
- Restless
- Pale or cyanotic

Palpation may reveal:
- Rapid, weak peripheral pulses
- Hepatomegaly in upper abdominal quadrant

Percussion may detect:
- Flatness over a widened area of the anterior chest

Auscultation may reveal:
- Decreased arterial blood pressure
- Pulsus paradoxus on inspiration
- Narrow pulse pressure
- Muffled heart sounds
- Clear lung fields

ATHOPHYSIOLOGY

Cardiac tamponade occurs when fluid or blood accumulates in the pericardial sac, thus reducing ventricular filling and cardiac output. The sac may stretch to allow for a slow pericardial effusion, and symptoms may not be apparent for some time. In acute accumulation, this results in cardiogenic shock and can be fatal if untreated.

Chapter 34. Ventricular Aneurysm

▽   ▽   ▽   ▽   ▽   ▽   ▽

INTRODUCTION

SEE TEXT PAGES

Ventricular aneurysm occurs when a necrotic area of the myocardium thins, forming a section of noncontracting ventricular wall.

SUPPORTING ASSESSMENT DATA

If your assessment findings are similar to those listed here, they may suggest ventricular aneurysm.

Health History:

In addition to the health risk factors listed in Chapter 7, "Coronary Artery Disease," consider at risk patients who have a history of the following:
• Myocardial infarction (MI)
• Angina
• Arrhythmias
• Palpitations

Physical Findings:

Patients with ventricular aneurysm are likely to complain of the following symptoms:
• Angina-like chest pain
• Fatigue
• Dyspnea

AMBULATORY CARE

When you assess an ambulatory patient who has a ventricular aneurysm, ask these questions:
• Have you ever had surgery to repair your heart aneurysm?
• Have you ever had a heart attack?
• Do you have a history of arrhythmias?
• Do you take Coumadin or aspirin?
• Do you wear a medical alert identification?

ASSESSMENT TECHNIQUES

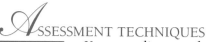

You may discover the following symptoms upon inspection:
- Visible precordial bulge
- Distended neck veins

You may discover the following symptoms upon palpation:
- Irregular peripheral pulses (see Chapter 9, "Myocardial Infarction")
- Pulsus alternans (see Chapter 32, "Cardiac Arrhythmias and Conduction Disturbances")
- Double, diffuse apical impulse, point of maximal impulse displaced

You may discover the following symptoms upon auscultation:
- Irregular rhythm
- Gallop rhythm
- Pulmonary crackles
- Pulmonary rhonchi

DIAGNOSTIC TESTS

TEST	FINDINGS
Chest X-ray	Bulge in heart **!** **NURSE ALERT:** Chest X-ray will appear normal if the aneurysm is small.
12-Lead ECG	• Rounded, ST-segment elevation over aneurysm location • ST shows T-wave elevations
Left ventriculography	• Enlarged left ventricle • Dyskinesia or akinesia • Reduced cardiac function
Echocardiography (2-D)	Abnormal left ventricular wall motion
Nuclear cardiology scan (noninvasive)	• Infarction • Aneurysm site

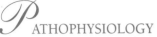ATHOPHYSIOLOGY

Ventricular aneurysm generally follows MI and usually occurs in the left ventricle.

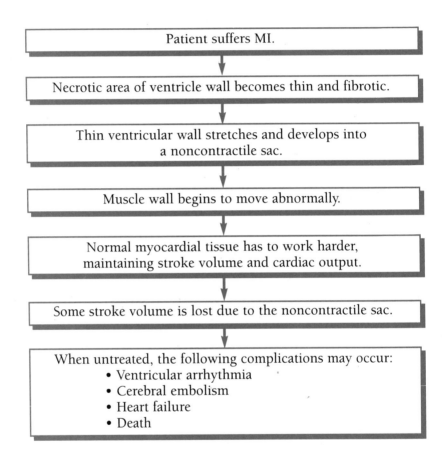

Patient suffers MI.

Necrotic area of ventricle wall becomes thin and fibrotic.

Thin ventricular wall stretches and develops into a noncontractile sac.

Muscle wall begins to move abnormally.

Normal myocardial tissue has to work harder, maintaining stroke volume and cardiac output.

Some stroke volume is lost due to the noncontractile sac.

When untreated, the following complications may occur:
- Ventricular arrhythmia
- Cerebral embolism
- Heart failure
- Death

Suggested Readings

Dreifus, L. S., et al. "Symptomatic Arrhythmias." *Patient Care* 26 (November 15, 1992): 176–190.

Fabius, D. B. "Diagnosing and Treating Ventricular Tachycardia," *Journal of Cardiovascular Nursing* 7 (April 1993): 8–25.

McGhie, A. I., and R. A.. Goldstein. "Parthenogenesis and Management of Acute Heart Failure and Cardiogenic Shock: Role of Inotropic Therapy," *Chest: The Cardiopulmonary Journal* 102 (November 1992): 626S–632S supplement.

Moore, K. "Do You Know These New Emergency Protocols?" *RN* 55 (1992): 34–35.

O'Neal, P. V. "How to Spot Early Signs of Cardiogenic Shock," *AJN* 94 (May 1994): 36–41.

Saver, C. L. "Decoding the ACLS Algorithms . . . Advanced Cardiac Life Support," *AJN* 94 (February 1994): 26–36.

Shoemaker, W. C. "Pathophysiology, Monitoring, and Therapy of Acute Circulatory Problems." *Critical Care Nursing Clinics of North America* 6 (June 1994): 295–307.

INDEX

J

Jugular veins, inspecting, 84
Junctional rhythm
   ECG criteria for, 224
   precipitating factors for, 217
Junctional tachycardia. See also
      Cardiac arrhythmias.
   ECG criteria for, 225
   precipitating factors for, 218

K

Kussmaul's respiration, pattern of, 41

L

Lower extremities, 66-68, 88
Lungs, auscultating, 94-95
Lymph nodes, assessing, 42

M

Male reproductive system, assessing,
      17
Mean arterial pressure, 75
Medical history, 79-80
Medication history, 80
Mitral insufficiency, 141-144
   diagnostic tests for, 143
   health history in, 141, 142
   pathophysiology of, 144
   physical findings in, 141
   signs and symptoms of, 142-143

Mitral stenosis, 137-140
   diagnostic tests for, 139
   health history in, 137, 138
   pathophysiology of, 139
   physical findings in, 137, 138
   progression of, 140
Mitral valve, 72
Mitral valve prolapse, chest pain in,
      81
Mouth and throat, assessing, 14,
      46-49
Musculoskeletal system, assessing,
      19-20
Myocardial infarction, 111-118
   chest pain in, 81
   diagnostic tests for, 113-114
   health history in, 111, 112
   pathophysiology of, 117
   physical findings in, 112
   signs and symptoms of, 112-113
   sites of, 117, 118
   trigger locations for, 115-116
Myocarditis, 181-182
   diagnostic tests for, 182
   health history in, 181
   pathophysiology of, 182
   physical findings in, 181
   signs and symptoms of, 182
Myocardium, 70

N

Nails, assessing, 12
Nasoscope, uses of, 30
Neck veins, inspecting, 84
Neurologic system, assessing, 19
Nose, assessing, 14, 45-46
Nutrition, assessing, 23

S

Order Other Titles In This Series!

Instant Nursing Assessment:

▲ Cardiovascular   0-8273-7102-0

▲ Respiratory   0-8273-7099-7

▲ Neurologic   0-8273-7103-9

▲ Women's Health   0-8273-7100-4

▲ Gerontologic   0-8273-7101-2

▲ Mental Health   0-8273-7104-7

▲ Pediatric   0-8273-7098-9

Rapid Nursing Interventions

▲ Cardiovascular   0-8273-7105-5

▲ Respiratory   0-8273-7095-4

▲ Neurologic   0-8273-7093-8

▲ Women's Health   0-8273-7092-X

▲ Gerontologic   0-8273-7094-6

▲ Mental Health   0-8273-7096-2

▲ Pediatric   0-8273-7097-0

- (cut here) -

Get "Instant" Experience!

QTY.	TITLE / ISBN	PRICE	TOTAL
		19.95	
		19.95	
		19.95	
		19.95	
		19.95	
		19.95	
	SUBTOTAL		
	STATE OR LOCAL TAXES		
	TOTAL		

Payment Information

☐ A Check is Enclosed

☐ Charge my ☐ VISA ☐ Mastercard   CARD # _____

MAIL OR FAX COMPLETED FORM TO:
Delmar Publishers • P.O. Box 15015 • Albany, NY 12212-5015

NAME _____

SCHOOL/INSTITUTION _____

STREET ADDRESS _____

CITY/STATE/ZIP _____

HOME PHONE _____

OFFICE PHONE _____

IN A HURRY TO ORDER? FAX: 1-518-464-0301
OR CALL TOLL-FREE 1-800-347-7707